Contents

Allied Health Professions – Essential Guides

Key Topics in Healthcare Management

Understanding the big picture

Edited by

Robert Jones

and

Fiona Jenkins

Series Foreword by
Penny Humphris

Foreword by
Professor Gerry McSorley

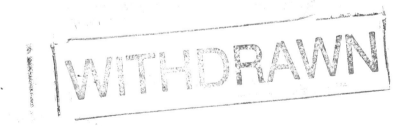

Radcliffe Publishing

Radcliffe Publishing Ltd
18 Marcham Road
Abingdon
Oxon OX14 1AA
United Kingdom

www.radcliffe-oxford.com
Electronic catalogue and worldwide online ordering facility.

British Library Cataloguing in Publication Data

A catalogue record for this book is available from the British Library.

ISBN-13: 978 1 85775 708 8

Typeset by Phoenix Photosetting, Chatham, Kent
Printed and bound by TJI Digital, Padstow, Cornwall

List of figures

List of tables

List of boxes

Series foreword

The NHS, the biggest organisation in the UK and reputedly the third largest in the world, is undergoing massive transformation. We know that effective leadership is essential if the health service is to achieve continuous improvement in the services it offers. It needs people from all types of backgrounds – clinical and managerial – to step up and take on leadership roles to shape the future of health improvement and healthcare delivery.

Leaders are needed at every level of the health service. The concept of leadership only coming from the top and being defined by position and title is now out of date. It is much more about ways of thinking and behaving and individuals seeing themselves as having the potential to make a real difference for patients. Effective leadership is about working in partnerships and teams to develop a vision for the future, set the direction, influence those whose input is needed and deliver results – a high quality, safe, timely and accessible health service for all.

Allied health professionals operate in every setting in which healthcare is delivered. You have unparalleled opportunities to help patients to lead their own care and to see how services to patients, clients and carers can be improved across entire patient pathways, crossing traditional professional and organisational boundaries to improve patients' experiences. You have the potential to make a difference by leading improvement and managing services and resources well.

There are already many outstanding leaders in the NHS in the allied health professions making a real difference to services. Two of them had the vision for this series of books and have worked with formidable energy and commitment to make them a reality. Robert and Fiona have both made a considerable investment in their own professional and personal development and delivered substantial improvements in the services for which they are responsible. They have increased their awareness, skills and knowledge and taken on leadership roles, putting into practice many of their ideas and learning. They have worked tirelessly to spread their learning and skilfully persuaded a great many academics and practitioners to contribute to these books to provide a rich collection of theories, tools, techniques and insights to help you.

This series of books has been written to encourage and support many more of you to embark on or to continue your development, to enhance your leadership and management skills, knowledge and experience and to give you confidence to take on new roles and responsibilities. I am sure that many of you, who have not previously considered yourselves as leaders will, when you have read these books, reconsider your roles and potential and take the next steps on your journeys.

Penny Humphris CBE
Former Director, NHS Leadership Centre
August 2007

Foreword

Capturing in writing the essence of good leadership and management is no small task. So much of what we observe, experience, share and witness of our actions and others' can be difficult to translate into text. As Levinson, a writer on leadership said some ten years ago 'Leadership is like beauty; it's hard to define, but you know it when you see it!' It is here that Rob Jones and Fiona Jenkins make such a mark. By compiling a series of experts who have translated the contemporary leadership, management and policy challenges into an excellent body of work to aid those committed to improving the standards of care to patients through their good management practice. Their collective efforts make for a journey of understanding and knowledge of great value to the reader in terms of the task of managing within the complex policy framework the NHS operates in today.

This complexity of policy and management is unlikely to become simpler with time. All agree that the shifting sands of politics, public and staff expectations will not, and arguably should not, stand still as we hope for better services. The movement to expansive careers and changing roles highlights the enormous contribution that Allied Health Professionals (AHPs) have to help drive forward the many improvements we all wish for. The need for continuing professional development is essential if this contribution is to be made to the full. Seizing the precious opportunity for critical thinking and reflection in otherwise busy lives will be greatly aided by the writing contained here.

The NHS is not short of space for great talent to come forward in small or large ways and AHPs continue to offer a unique clinical viewpoint on how we enrich the way we design and deliver healthcare. It is through our shared understanding of the climate we work in and the techniques of good management and self-reflection that drive on our vocation, that our hopes and aspirations for progress will be gained.

Jaworski highlights the key attribute of leadership (either in us or in others) as about creating the domain in which we continually learn and become more capable of participating in our unfolding future. He argues that we must shift from seeing the world as clockwork, fixed and machinelike, to one which is open, dynamic and interconnected, and full of living qualities. Once we see this shift we move from resignation to a sense of possibility. We are then able to create the future every moment.

Jones and Jenkins, along with their co-writers, provide such a sense of possibility and therefore an impressive step to a better future.

Gerry McSorley
Honorary President, Institute of Healthcare Management
August 2007

Preface

There are many challenges and opportunities for healthcare managers; the NHS reform agenda and the multi-layered strategy for service improvement is extensive and complex. AHPs are well placed to make significant and positive contributions to the provision of effective and efficient, patient-centred and responsive services. The many challenges and opportunities should be used to stimulate action, thought, reflective practice and innovation in service provision and we hope that the scope, spectrum and depth of chapters in this book will be supportive.

There are many publications available on all aspects of management theory and practice. However, to date there has not been a specific book focusing on the key 'Big Picture' topics as they relate in particular to the Allied Health Professions. With so many fundamental and radical changes and upheavals taking place at such a rapid pace in the NHS and health services worldwide, we believe that this is the right time for this book to set out and expand on the broad context of change and development in healthcare management, leadership and development.

Our series 'Allied Health Professions – Essential Guides', of which this is the third book, is intended for AHP managers and aspiring managers, leaders, clinicians, researchers, educators, students and non-AHP Registrants within the remit of the Health Professions Council. The series is also useful for doctors, nurses, pharmacists, optometrists, other professionals working in healthcare management and leadership roles and general managers.

This volume focuses on the context of structural, organisational and management changes within the NHS and wider health and social care environments, encompassing theory and practice, policy developments, innovations and new or different ways of working. The areas explored and discussed relate to the NHS and wider healthcare provision in the 21st century. The perspective is wide ranging focusing on important broad vision issues which are all parts of the overall picture and about which – we believe – managers and leaders need an understanding in order to work effectively and succeed.

All of the contributors to this volume, *Key Topics in Healthcare Management – understanding the big picture,* have recognised expertise nationally and internationally and are widely experienced in their fields. The text is not a continuous narrative, but a collection of subjects closely related and linked into the whole to provide a comprehensive view of the context, content and relevance of issues which overarch many areas; all topics relevant to the development, provision and maintenance of 'best quality' services for patients, clients and service users. We have not attempted to significantly adjust the style of individual authors, although each chapter stands in its own right, there are major themes which bring the different aspects together.

We would like to thank all of our contributors for sharing their knowledge, experience and expertise, it was a great privilege to work in close collaboration and harmony with them all. We would also like to thank our publisher, Radcliffe Publishing Ltd for their support, encouragement and expertise.

AHPs must be proactive and responsive to the many changes taking place, whenever and wherever possible, to see the upheavals as opportunities, transforming them into positive steps towards the improvement of our services. There is no 'best, right or only one way' of management and leadership; our aim, and that of all our contributors, is to set out approaches and provide an in-depth and wide range of information which we believe will enhance the evidence-base, knowledge, understanding and skills to support managers, leaders and clinicians to manage and lead their services pro-actively, effectively and efficiently and by so doing, provide the best quality service possible for our patients and service users.

Robert Jones and Fiona Jenkins
August 2007
www.jjconsulting.org.uk

About the editors

Dr Robert Jones PhD, M.Phil, BA, FCSP, Grad Dip Phys, MHSM, MMACP
Head of Therapy Services, East Sussex Hospitals NHS Trust.

Robert has management responsibility for therapy services in one of the largest trusts in the country. He manages a large team of therapy and support staff in acute services, primary care, external contracts and the independent sector.

A Physiotherapist by background, he is the former Physiotherapy Registrant Member of the HPC and a former Chair and Vice President of the Chartered Society of Physiotherapy.

Robert was seconded to the Commission for Health Improvement for a year as AHP consultant/advisor, he represented AHPs on the NHS Information Authority Project Board and QAA steering group. He lectures both nationally and internationally on management topics, IM&T in Allied Health Professions and service improvement and design. His PhD is in management and his M.Phil is in Social Policy, he has published widely on management and clinical topics.

Fiona Jenkins MA (dist.), FCSP, Grad Dip Phys, MHSM, NEBS Dip(M), PGCO
Non-medical Clinical Director of Therapy Services, South Devon Healthcare Foundation Trust.

Fiona manages a physiotherapy service in a large acute trust with services also provided in primary care. A former Council member and Vice President of the Chartered Society of Physiotherapy, Fiona has led a large number of service improvements across South Devon which have received national recognition. She lectures both nationally and internationally on management topics. Her MA is in management, and she is currently further undertaking research for a PhD.

Fiona and Robert successfully completed the INSEAD NHS/Leadership Centre Clinical Strategists' programme at the business school in Fontainebleau Paris and continue to undertake project work with the university. They were Modernisation Agency Associates and have worked collaboratively on service improvements, developments and innovation. They have established a consultancy, which provides management workshops, masterclasses, lectures and presentations on healthcare management topics nationally and internationally: www.jjconsulting.org.uk.

List of contributors

Helen Anderson BA, FCIPD
Human Resources Consultant, London

Professor Rosalie A Boyce PhD, Mbus, BSc, Grad Dip Dietetic,
Grad Dip Health Admin
School of Pharmacy, University of Queensland
Visiting Professor, Sheffield Hallam University

Dr Sally French PhD, MSc (Psych), MSc (Soc), BSc, Dip TP, MCSP
Associate Lecturer Open University

Professor Alan Gillies PhD, MA, MILT, MUKCHIP, Doctor Honoris Causa
Professor in Information Management
University of Central Lancashire

Dr Gail Louw PhD, MA, MSc, BA
Principal Lecturer
Institute of Postgraduate Medicine
Brighton and Sussex Medical School

Laura McDonnell BSc (Hons)
Stress Programme Team
HSE
Health and Work Division
London

Dr Anne Mandy PhD, MSc, BSc (Hons), Cert Ed
Research Student Division Leader
Principal Research Fellow
Clinical Research Centre
University of Brighton

Dr Sharon Mickan PhD, MA, BOT (Aust), Cert Ed
Consultant Researcher, University of Queensland
Mickan Consulting, Frankfurt and Brisbane

Dr Patricia Oakley PhD (Organisational Psychology), MBA (London),
BSc (Pharmacy), Grad IPD, MRPharmS, DHMSA
Director, Practices Made Perfect Ltd
London
www.practices.co.uk

Tove Steen Sørensen-Bentham MSc, Llm
Principal Lecturer
Brighton Business School, University of Brighton

Claire Sullivan MA, MCSP, Grad Dip Phys
Assistant Director of Employment Relations and Union Services
Chartered Society of Physiotherapy
London

Professor John Swain PhD, MSc, BSc, PGCE
Professor of Disability and Inclusion
University of Northumbria

List of abbreviations

A&E	Accident and Emergency
ACAS	Advisory, Conciliation and Arbitration Service
ACEVO	Association of Chief Executives of Voluntary Organisations
ACOP	Approved Codes of Practice
AfC	Agenda for Change
AHP	Allied Health Profession
AHPs	Allied Health Profession(s)
BDA	British Dietetic Association
BIOS	British Orthoptic Society
BMA	British Medical Association
BPR	Business Process re-engineering
CEO	Chief Executive Officer
CHAI	Commission for Healthcare Audit and Inspection
CHI	Commission for Health Improvement
CMO	Chief Medical Officer
CNST	Clinical Negligence Scheme for Trusts
COT	College of Occupational Therapists
COSHH	Control of Substances Hazardous to Health
CPD	Continuing Professional Development
CSP	Chartered Society of Physiotherapy
CT	Computer Tomography
DDA	Disability Discrimination Act
DET	Disability Equality Training
DH	Department of Health
DoH	Department of Health
DHSS	Department of Health and Social Security
DNA	Did Not Attend
DSE	Display Screen Equipment
E-mail	Electronic Mail
EPP	Expert Patient Programme
EU	European Union
EWTD	European Working Time Directive
GMC	General Medical Council
GMS	General Medical Services
GP	General Practitioner
HASAWA	Health and Safety at Work Act
HMSO	Her Majesty's Stationery Office
HPC	Health Professions Council
HR	Human Resources
HRM	Human Resource Management
HSC	Health and Safety Commission
HSE	Health and Safety Executive

ICP	Integrated care pathway
IIP	Investors in People
IM&T	Information Management and Technology
ISO	International Standards Organisation
IT	Information Technology
IWL	Improving Working Lives
KSF	Knowledge and Skills Framework
NHS	National Health Service
NHSLA	National Health Service Litigation Authority
NHSNI	National Health Service Northern Ireland
NICE	National Institute for Health and Clinical Excellence
NMC	Nursing and Midwifery Council
NPA	National Pathways Association
NRLS	National Reporting and Learning System
NSF	National Service Framework
OECD	Organisation for Economic Co-operation and Development
PBC	Practice Based Commissioning
PbR	Payment by Results
PCRN	Primary Care Research Network
PCT	Primary Care Trust
PDSA	Plan Do Study Act
PEST	Political Economic Social and Technological
PMETB	Post Graduate Medical Education and Training Board
PPI	Patient and Public Involvement
QOF	Quality Outcomes Framework
RCSLT	Royal College of Speech and Language Therapist
SCP	Society of Chiropodists and Podiatrists
SFI	Standing Financial Instructions
SHA	Strategic Health Authority
SMART	Specific Measurable Achievable Realistic Timed
SNDMSG	Send Message
SOR	Society of Radiographers
SS	Social Services
SWOT	Strengths, Weaknesses, Opportunities, Threats
RIDDOR	Reporting of Injuries, Diseases and Dangerous Occurrences Regulations
TIA	Transient Ischaemic Attack
TQM	Total Quality Management
TUC	Trades Union Congress
UK	United Kingdom
USA	United States of America
VDU	Visual Display Unit
www	World Wide Web

List of books in this series

Public policy reforms and the National Health Service strategic development agenda

Patricia Oakley

Introduction

A dynamic Public Policy Reform agenda

As an illustration of the dynamic situation; at the time of writing, for instance, the Government is working on complex legislation and major proposals to:

- reform the way in which medical and professional staff are going to be reaccredited and validated in the future during all of their working lives
- develop public service commissioning in the NHS, the secondary education service, and the prison and probation services, which will have a bearing on how therapy services will be developed in the future
- build up the intriguingly titled '3rd sector' as a supplementary provider of public services which will affect future models of care provision.

Within this changing environment, the aim of this chapter is to pinpoint the key policy areas which are now fairly stable features of the Public Policy Reform Agenda so that Allied Health Professions (AHPs) Managers can start to see more clearly how their AHP services will be commissioned, provided, and quality assured in the future. To this end, this chapter represents a synthesis of much research which has been augmented by the Author's practice in many streams of policy and development work across the public sector. Parts of this chapter have appeared in earlier forms in various working papers, policy masterclasses and their supporting notes, and service evaluation reports for clients especially over the last five years.

The context for developing AHP services in the 21st century

There are at least five important forces which are driving the development of AHP services in the 21st century:

1 the changing population profile and people's needs as they live longer in a more independent way while being increasingly sensitive to the tax burden

2   the desire to achieve a more 'joined-up' approach to public service policy-making, service commissioning and its provision, with the desired collective effect of achieving 'improved outcomes'

3   the desire to achieve a more locally accountable government structure in the form of devolution to the Regional Assembly Governments in Wales, Scotland, Northern Ireland and London, and possibly – in time – to the other English regions

4   the changing legal context being driven by shifts in European law, for example in employment practices and the free movement of labour across member states, and in clinical practices and the conduct of safer and more rigorous clinical trials

5   The changing risk management environment as a result of major inquiries and legal rulings clarifying and assigning duties and responsibilities.

Taking the first point to locate this introductory discussion in AHP services, within the last ten years, there have been several major reports on people's changing needs for health and social care including:

- the Report of the Royal Commission on Long Term Care, 1999[1]
- the Audit Commission's series of reports[2,3,4,5,6] covering health and social care provision, 1997–2000
- the Department of Health (DH) proposals to improve chronic disease management.[7,8]

These reports, and many others, have explained why, and informed how, AHP services should be delivered in a more integrated way focusing on chronic disease management with an emphasis on self-care and the provision of intermediate care. The comparative review by Ham *et al*[9] of hospital bed utilisation in the NHS with the US Kaiser Permanente and Medicare Programmes in 2003 gives an initial analysis of the data to support this proposition.

The other driving forces will be discussed in the relevant sections below.

The structure of this chapter

This chapter also discusses Government policies in a hierarchical analysis which covers:

- an overview of the Public Service Reform Agenda to show the common ideas emerging across the public service so the NHS reforms can be located in the wider policy context
- an overview of the NHS commissioning reforms including the development of the more aggregated primary care trusts (PCTs) in England and their equivalents in the devolved administrations
- an overview of the NHS provider organisations including the social enterprises and voluntary sector which make up the '3rd sector' and the changing regulatory structure which affects the workforce.

The chapter concludes with an assessment of the potential collective impact of these reforms on developing AHP services in the 21st century and it offers AHP managers a 'watch list' of key issues which they will need to address in order to reform their services.

The public service reform agenda

Developing commissioning and providing

The public service reform agenda emphasises the separation of service commissioning from its provision. For example, in social services, which have operated this policy for many years, the White Paper for England,[10] sought to further integrate health and social care provision, and to develop more integrated service commissioning for care of the elderly and for those with long-term conditions. Similarly, the Government's proposed reform of the provision of secondary schools in England will result in the Local Education Authorities becoming in time, commissioners of secondary education and secondary schools developing in a more independent and plural way driven by local demands.[11]

The Government also proposes a major reform of its prison and probation services (for England and Wales) following the Carter Review.[12] This in effect follows the pattern above but requires new and complex legal powers to develop 'Correctional Services' commissioning, through a new body called the National Offender Management Service, and a more integrated prison and probation service which focuses on providing prisoners with bespoke rehabilitation and treatment programmes so that their resettlement in the community is likely to be more successful. Currently, up to 60% of discharged prisoners reoffend and return to prison within one to two years of their discharge date. Critically, much of the rehabilitation and treatment programmes required consist of education and skills building supported by mental health and detoxification treatment programmes.

In addition, in respect of the 'Lifers' and those detained indefinitely in the specialist psychiatric prisons, the Government proposes a programme of support as these prisoners become old and infirm, and suffer from the normal process of ageing including senile dementia. Because the reform programme is so complex and sensitive, it will take a number of years to implement but clearly there are overlaps between the programme commissioners for correctional services and the emerging commissioning roles for the education, health and social services.[13,14]

'Choice' and patient power

The 'choice' agenda reflects in part the shifting public attitudes to public service provision, especially in England. This is illustrated by two contrasting populations of mature and elderly women. On the one hand, is a group of women born after World War Two – the 'baby boomers' who are relatively more educated, especially as a result of the education reforms that took effect in the mid to late 1960s and who have had jobs resulting in pension contributions and savings over a long working life. This group forms the next generation of women pensioners who are in effect 'healthier, stealthier and wealthier'. They have different attitudes to public service provision which they have contributed to for all their working lives and they tend to be well-informed 'consumers'.

In contrast, there is a group of women pensioners who have experienced the horrors and deprivations of life before and during the Second World War and who saw the birth of the NHS and its universal 'free' service. They tend to be less 'muscular' in asserting their rights. With an emphasis on looking after themselves and their family, mature and elderly women form the backbone of the UK carer 'workforce', and they are critical to the well-being of not just themselves but also of their families. In policy terms, the Government needs to satisfy both groups to prevent a two-tier service emerging. For brevity, this is a gross simplification of the social group mixes as the story is indeed much more complex. However, this brief explanation underpins, in part, the Government's proposals to develop under the aegis of the White Paper, the 'Expert Patient' Programme, focusing on Long Term Conditions such as diabetes, mental health, cardiac problems.[8] In addition, there are about four million people in the UK in receipt of disability benefits. The Government seeks to mobilise a proportion of these people back into the workplace under the 'Pathways to Work' scheme.[15] As a result, they will require support for their Long Term Conditions, particularly mental health problems.[16]

With the growth in the proportion of the elderly in the UK, and the commensurate pressure on the tax-funded health and social care service, and an increasingly tax-averse public, the policy bundle described above needs to be supported by an expanded service and therefore more resources. The proposals to bring health and social care closer together opens the public debate about funding a future joint service and the issue of whether the Government should allow more direct and co-payments which are used in social services to support the directly funded service from the taxpayer. This is a major policy issue for the next general election.

Developing the market

The Government has developed a number of policy instruments to underpin the proposed market system which will operate in England. Two central developments are the framework of rules to make the market work which is known as the contestability process, and the introduction of foundation NHS trusts. As NHS trusts meet the strict financial performance criteria, they are granted such status which in effect loosens them up from some central control making them a little more independent, but accountable to the public service commissioner.

To support the market, the Government is developing a set of tables which state the 'programme of care and its tariff'. At the moment, it covers England only, mainly in surgical procedures but there are plans to bring out similar tables for programmes covering long-term conditions and mental health services in 2006–09. Once the glitches have been resolved, and the proposed contract currencies are validated, this will allow the market to operate from about 2008–09. It is complicated work and it is estimated that it will take 10–15 years to bed down in the NHS (based on experiences in the US and Germany).

To develop the market in England, the Government needs to protect the taxpayer and patients. To this end, it has set up a Market Regulator – known in the NHS as Monitor – which has powers of entry to foundation trusts if they deviate from their financial tolerance levels when it can issue painful course correction notices. The Government has also set up an inspectorate known as the Health Commissioner who has power of entry to the whole service on a rolling basis of inspection when it can issue improvement notices and recommendations for change. The Government also needs a Contract Compliance Officer who can ensure the performance of the contracts issued by the Service Commissioner. This office is likely to be located in the new – Regional – Strategic Health Authorities (SHAs) (see discussion below). In practice, these roles have some degree of overlap and following a review, the Government will clarify their future domains of authority.

Developing service commissioning and accountability

Strengthening financial governance and accountability

The Government raises taxes from the British public and allocates the resources against the many claims on the fund after Parliament has approved the Government's budget. Part of this fund is then allocated to the Scottish Parliament, Welsh Assembly Government and the Northern Ireland Office and their First Ministers, elected members and lead officers decide how much of their fund will be spent on the NHS within their jurisdiction. In England, the fund for the NHS is allocated to the DH which then administers it through the SHAs.

As it is public money, it has to be accounted for to Parliament where the Comptroller and Auditor General reports on the value for money achieved and the efficiency of the public service. Similar arrangements apply in the devolved administrations. As a result of this strong financial governance framework, the NHS has to publicly allocate, and account for, its resources according to the rules laid out in the Standing Financial Orders, Standing Financial Instructions and the Scheme of Reservations and Delegations.[17]

Two important developments will affect how the financial governance and reporting framework will operate in the NHS in the future:

1 the Enron disaster and the Higgs Commission – as a result of the Enron financial disaster and subsequent inquiries in the US, the UK Government (via HM Treasury and the Department for Trade and Industry) commissioned a review of the likelihood that such a disaster could happen in the UK. The resulting Higgs Report has highlighted potential weaknesses particularly in the way Boards work in their scrutiny role and has made recommendations to strengthen this area. These recommendations inform how public bodies need to strengthen their financial governance arrangements[18]
2 the Arm's Length Bodies Review – to ensure that the bulk of taxpayers money is spent on public services rather than on an infrastructure of bureaucracy, the Government has started a review of all the Arm's Length Bodies with a view to reducing their numbers and size, and to streamlining the costs of administering public services. As a result, many inspection and advisory bodies, and public funding bodies, are being merged, or disbanded, and their running costs severely capped.[19]

This set of developments creates the context within which the NHS commissioning system will develop over the next three to five years.

NHS commissioning and accountability across the UK

A recent review of the effectiveness of primary care led commissioning and its place in the NHS from the Health Foundation has shown that from 1991–1997, commissioning policy was largely consistent across the four countries of the UK. Since 1997 however, the approach has varied, and the authors[20] have summarised this in Table 1.1.

Table 1.1 NHS commissioning.

England	the purchaser-provider split has been largely retained and PCTs have become the main local commissioning body and they are charged with developing new forms of devolved practice-led commissioning
Northern Ireland	local health and social groups have been created as a method of developing effective clinical and public engagement in the commissioning process. The groups have however struggled to secure GP involvement
Scotland	the quasi-market was abolished and the funding system was returned to the directly managed – central allocation system where commissioning and providing roles are effectively integrated. Community Health Partnerships are viewed as key forums for determining local health and social care priorities and plans
Wales	the purchaser-provider split has been retained with a strong emphasis on forming local partnerships with local Government and local communities focused on 22 Local Health Boards

Table 1.2 Changes in commissioning processes.

England	the number of SHAs and PCTs has been dramatically reduced and their respective roles and responsibilities are being redefined to focus them on developing more effective service commissioning and accountability. As a result, PCTs now cover larger geographical areas and they are supported by a number of administrative back up services which are organised at a regional level to achieve economies of scale savings. PCTs have a specific duty to develop GP practice-based commissioning and they will lose, in time, their service provider duties
Northern Ireland	the number of Health and Social Service Boards and their constituent Health and Social Care trusts has been dramatically reduced so that there is now one Board for Northern Ireland which will commission and work with five super health and social care provider organisations. It is unclear how GP involvement will be taken forward
Scotland	the number of Health Boards and their functions are under review and the development of service commissioning and performance management within the context of the local Community Health Partnerships depends on how the Scottish Parliament wants to develop its governance and accountability structures and processes, including involving GPs
Wales	the number of Local Health Boards, working with their local authority partners, is under review but many have already developed shared commissioning duties and responsibilities across three regional networks which are also supported by a national commissioning group

In the light of this discussion and the pressure to reduce administration costs while increasing the rigour of the NHS financial governance, there are a number of changes to the structures and processes of NHS commissioning across the UK, shown in Table 1.2.

Clearly, service commissioning across the UK is developing according to each country's culture and requirements and may be seen on a conceptual continuum of the level of market forces applied to create performance pressures in the providers, as shown in Figure 1.1.

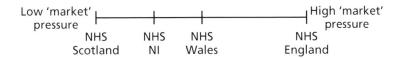

Figure 1.1 Market forces providing pressure for providers.

Developing commissioning in England

Service Commissioners across the UK commission the services that are required by their local populations as defined by the local Public Health Strategies which are based on careful local audits and research. Where possible, the commissioning plans are underpinned by evidence-based practices and much of these are informed by the standards laid down by the various august bodies such as the medical Royal Colleges and the National Standards Boards working across the UK.

In England, service commissioning needs to be organised where possible on a scaled basis to ensure the administrative costs are minimised. Therefore, where it is possible and sensible to do so, some services will be commissioned and quality assured on a national basis through the National Specialised Services Commissioning Group. For example, the transplant programmes, the specialist children's and orthopaedic services, and the medium- long-term secure mental health units, are all likely to be commissioned nationally.

Some services are already organised on a regional basis for example the intensivist and emergency services so they will probably be commissioned and quality assured on a regional – or even pan-regional basis. Similarly, there are a number of clinical networks which have the necessary expertise to commission and quality assure their services, for example in cancer and cardiology, so they might reasonably form the specialist commissioning groups.

GPs, working in consortia of practices, possibly organised on a locality basis, would seem to be a sensible place to locate the commissioning of long-term care services. As GPs are also providers of care, and subject to the service agreements and bonuses set out in the new General Medical Services (GMS) contract, the legal and financial details of GPs' roles as both commissioners and providers of the same service will need to be clarified and separated to avoid accusations of conflicts of interest and potentially risks to patients.

At the time of writing, the NHS for England is undergoing a major reorganisation so much of the above is still work in progress. However, although early days, the SHAs work programmes to implement the reforms is emerging. These are summarised in the Figure 1.2.

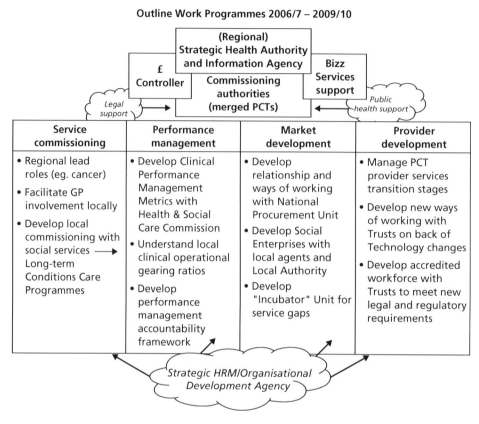

Figure 1.2 Developing commissioning and performance management and reforming the Primary Care Trusts in England.

In summary, the five part work programme probably includes the following:

1 build up the new merged regionally based SHAs and their support teams and agencies to provide financial, information and business support services, and possibly public health and legal services, for the merged PCTs as they develop their role as Commissioners

2 build up the service commissioning infrastructure by developing the commissioning and performance management roles and responsibilities of the clinical networks for specialist services, for example cancer, cardiology, and intensivist services; and similarly, facilitate and develop the consortia of GP practices to commission, with social services, programmes of care for those with long-term needs

3 build up the performance management programme including the underpinning clinical metrics, informatics, and methodology incorporating the work of the Health and Social Care Commission, the Royal Colleges and the Audit Commission

4 develop the market locally in partnership with the National Procurement Unit, which lets contracts for specialist clinical services such as primary care, imaging and surgical services; and with the Social Enterprise Unit, which facilitates, with local agents, the development of local community-based services. There

are probably going to be a few difficult or new, or 'orphaned' services which will need support to pilot and mature them so an 'incubator' unit will be required

5 manage the transition and develop the PCT's direct labour provider services, incorporating new ways of working and the new accreditation requirements (see below), and transfer them, in time, to the most appropriate provider organisation.

This complex and extensive work programme will require support from human resource management and organisational development specialists, possibly organised on a pan-commissioner or regional basis.

Developing service providers

Strategic development objectives of the policy

There are many challenges facing the NHS in the 21st century. In addition to the need to reduce the risks that patients potentially face, the NHS will need to address the following issues within the context of devolution:

• the pressure on service budgets as the Government seeks to reduce the size of the underlying deficits and increase the service's efficiency levels and effectiveness
• the requirement to build systemic quality assurance procedures into the clinical protocols that form the care pathway, especially concerning easy access to, and the best use of, information about the procedures and clinicians
• the requirement to develop effective multidisciplinary team working and shared responsibility for decision-making
• the pressure to address patients' and carers' choices, especially in England[21]
• the requirement to implement in some parts of the UK a new payment/cash allocation system, for example the Payment by Results Tariff in England.[22]

The next wave of NHS and social care reforms, building on previous changes within the context of devolution, have the following key policy objectives to:

• improve access to good quality acute and primary care services by reducing waiting times and building more patient-focused evidence-based programmes of care
• increase the service's efficiency and performance levels by improving the organisation and management of clinical care
• develop new ways of working to reduce bureaucracy, duplication and hold-ups in providing clinical services
• shift the NHS cost structure from the current fixed cost system to one which is more flexible and variable
• embed quality assurance and risk management within the service's design and ways of working.

In addition, the recently published White Paper proposes for England[10] the development of more integrated health and social care services provided outside hospitals and nearer to, or in, patients' own homes. It places emphasis on involving patients with long-term conditions, and their carers, in planning and providing for their own care through:

- learning about how to manage and live with their condition through the 'Expert' Patient Programme[8]
- purchasing packages of care directly from local approved suppliers using public funds allocated under the direct and co-payments scheme which was successfully piloted in England during the last Government
- having access to specialists locally, particularly for diagnostic tests and investigations, some procedures, and clinical services including surgery, gynaecology, ear, nose and throat, cancer care, some general medicine, urology and dermatology.

Developing a plurality of providers

To support the expansion and development of long-term care provision in the community, particularly in England, the Government has made available the following five legal formulations to underpin potential service providers so that they may be considered and included on the public procurement list for service commissioners:

1 public foundation trusts
2 public limited companies
3 registered charities
4 registered partnerships
5 social enterprises.

The details of these legal formulations are:

1 **public foundation trusts** are in their infancy in England but it seems likely that most NHS providers will be expected to meet the stricter financial and operational control requirements of such status by 2008, hence we may assume that most NHS provider organisations will have achieved foundation trust status by 2008– 09. At the moment, this applies to secondary care but the NHS Regulator for England is currently considering how this status might be applied to the community services provided currently under the aegis of PCTs
2 **public limited companies** are registered under the Companies Act and they have to meet the strict financial reporting requirements of this Act which may be enhanced soon in the light of the Enron disaster in the USA, and the subsequent Higgs Commission of Inquiry in the UK which has assessed the current potential risks of such financial impropriety occurring in UK registered companies. Much of the expanded health and social service provision in England over the last 10 years has been provided by registered companies, and this trend seems set to continue in the future
3 **registered charities** are registered under the Charities Act and they have to meet the strict financial reporting requirements of the Act which has been enhanced recently following a review of its fitness for purpose in the 21st century. Registered charities range from being very small local groups of individuals who are united around a heartfelt cause, such as providing educational support against the use of drugs in memory of a loved one who has died, to major multi-national complex organisations which provide specialised services, for example the Marie Curie Foundation and the Macmillan Nursing Service. Many of these charities enjoy high levels of recognition and respect amongst the public and their increasingly expanded

role in providing specialist health and social care services locally is expected to continue in the future

4 **registered partnerships** are owned by its founders who are called partners, and their organisations are registered under the Partnership Act which has been strengthened in the recent past to offer a form of limited liability following several major court cases brought against world-class accountancy firms. It is used as the legal formulation of choice to support the establishment of traditional GP services and this historical pattern is set to continue for the foreseeable future. However, this model of service provision might start to see a gradual decline as the current owners of registered GP practices retire and their successors use other legal formulations to support their health and social care enterprises

5 **social enterprises** are workers' co-operatives or mutual organisations set-up under a new legal form called the Community Interest Company. In its re-election Manifesto of May 2005, the Government made its commitment to such organisations clear by stating that it believed these organisations:

> have an important role to play in the provision of local services, from health to education, from leisure to care of the vulnerable … its potential for service delivery should be considered on equal terms.

Although early days, there have been several successful initiatives under this development in Northern Ireland and England. While such initiatives tend to be small at the moment, in England consideration is being given to commissioning a proposed pilot scheme to provide community-based nursing and therapy service involving nearly 800 staff from such a workers' co-operative. We do not know if the idea will stand the pressures associated with scale but given the Government's commitment in its manifesto, these types of organisation could increasingly provide community-based services.

Developing care outside hospitals

To support these proposed developments, the Government intends to commission for England at least 50 new community-based hospitals which might include diagnostic centres as well as consultation and treatment rooms and facilities for providing rehabilitation and AHP services.

Looking to the future, it is likely, especially in England, that the expanded service provider map will be much more plural in nature. This is summarised in the diagram below which distinguishes on the one hand the location of future services in the high street and the hospital campuses, and on the other, services which are supported by low-technology or ultra high-technology.

These major developments in the provision of community-based care in England are being mirrored by complementary developments in the devolved administrations, for example in Wales, under 'Designed for Life', which builds on the recommendations of the Wanless Report for Wales,[23] and in Scotland, NHS Scotland seeks to address its major public health agenda – tobacco, cancer, food and health, sexual health, physical activity, mental health, drug misuse, alcohol problems, health inequalities – by community-based policy developments within each of its 15 Boards working with their local authorities, to achieve the objectives set out in 'Delivering for Health'.[24] Clearly, each administration will develop its

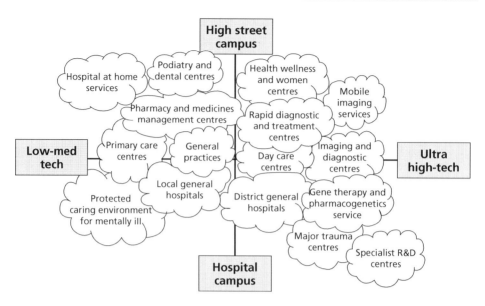

Figure 1.3 Developing a plurality of providers – the component services.

own policies and ways of working to meet the challenges it faces but the broad direction of travel seems to be based on the following generic policies:

- the development of some GP practices into providing more specialised services under the aegis of the GMS contract and the Quality and Outcomes Framework (QOF)
- the development of community pharmacy services under the Medicines Management Initiative and the new General Pharmacy Services Contract
- the development of community nursing services under the 'Community Matrons' initiative and the strategy for advanced nursing practice development
- the development of the ambulance trusts' paramedical services and the upgrading of the paramedics' 'first responder' skills and ways of working
- the development of accredited prescribers who can both initiate, in some cases, and maintain AHP services under the aegis of a medical practitioner.

Developing multi-agency cinical networks

In a parallel set of policy developments, the Government and the Devolved Administrations, building on earlier policies to encourage partnership working between providers in public agencies, has encouraged the development of managerial and financial convergence in such partnerships. Under a lead chief officer, who is accountable to a number of public bodies that form the multi-agency network, the three key services that are affected by this policy are:

1 children's care services
2 mental healthcare services
3 care of the elderly services.

This pattern of networking several organisations and bringing together their planning and financial standing orders to form a coherent virtual whole organisation fixed on a care group has been replicated with varying degrees of success in the following clinical services:

- cancer and cardiology networks
- surgical and intensive care networks
- emergency services networks.

The longer term success of this bridging device between NHS organisations which provide either primary or secondary care services is not known but the Department of Health for England has commissioned a major review of the clinical networking programme, and the pilot multi-agency partnerships, to assess if they will be substantiated beyond 2008 when the current support funding finishes.

Developing a network of emergency and unplanned care services

The network is an effective inter-organisational development tool to support the changes required in three key interrelated services:

1 emergency care networks
2 surgical service networks
3 intensivist care networks.

Currently, these services are organised in relatively discrete pockets within the District General Hospitals and the major teaching hospitals. They are supported by the GP out-of-hours service and the ambulance trusts. There are unique pressures in each of these highly specialised services which when taken together give the rationale for reforming and reorganising emergency and unplanned care services.

1 **Emergency care networks**: Accident and Emergency Departments (A&E) are well recognised and used by the public as a safe port of call for most of their problems especially when the other statutory agencies are shut. As a result, over the years, these departments have built up their services and 'know-how' in distinct areas:

- trauma services which can form about 1–2% of the work for most departments
- minor injuries which can form about two-thirds of the workload
- major injuries which can form the balance of the work.

Staffing such specialist services with accredited competent individuals around the clock in rota and shift patterns that comply with the increasingly tight regulations is getting more difficult. Therefore, local health communities are looking at ways of reorganising the work flows and making better use of the resources available. As a result, local emergency care networks are being developed which seek to integrate the discrete components into a more coherent 'whole' multi-agency service. The resulting more focused deployment of skills and clarified relationships gives a potential four level organisational network structure for the service.[4,5,6,7,8] This network is summarised in Figure 1.4.

2 **Surgical services networks**: at the same time, surgical services are becoming increasingly specialised[25,26,27,28] and some surgeons' and anaesthetists' ability to cross-cover in other general areas is becoming more difficult as they will need to be accredited as competent in those areas in the future as the regulations

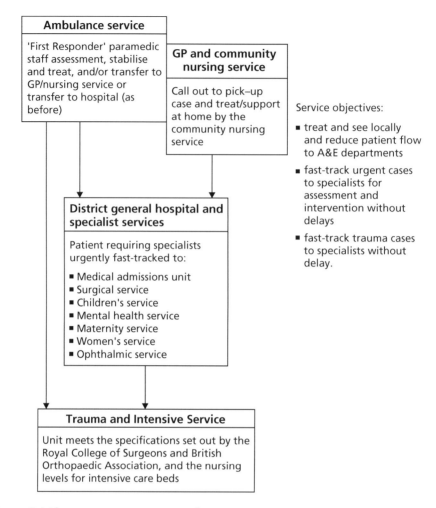

Figure 1.4 The emergency care network.

become tighter. This creates pressure on the smaller and mid-sized district general hospitals in particular as their 'pool' of accredited staff is relatively smaller so that ultimately they cannot meet the new rota and shifts for the accident and emergency departments as they might have done in the past. This pressure is exacerbated by the historical shifts that have been taking place over the last 20 years and the current trends to:

- concentrate specialist surgical services in centres of excellence, such as neurosurgery, cardiology, urology, cancer, ophthalmology, paediatrics
- concentrate elective surgery in centres of excellence for example orthopaedics, and transfer some cases to private sector units in England
- increase the proportion of day case surgery including the transfer of some cases to private sector units in England.

The net result is that patients and their GPs and community nurses will need access to a range of hospitals and specialist services, and this may mean that for some specialist services, patients – and their carers – may have to travel further afield.

3 **Intensivist care networks**: to complement the developments outlined above, the intensivist care networks[29] are increasingly forming around the patient's level of critical illness in a four level system as illustrated in Figure 1.5.

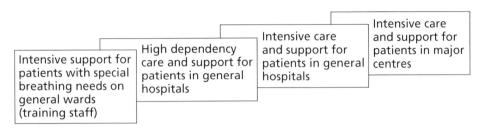

Figure 1.5 The intensivist care network.

This local networking creates a supportive environment for potentially isolated services. In some cases however, as the staffing levels are very high for example in intensive care units, at least six qualified intensivist nurses are required for each bed, maintaining the provision of such services is increasingly difficult in some local general hospitals. Without this crucial back-up service, local A&E departments and surgical services cannot be maintained.

Developing a multiplicity of 'hospitals'

The challenge of this collective pressure is forcing trusts to work together to find an acceptable resolution to these complex issues. It will mean that in the future, local health communities will be more interdependent as specialist services are concentrated in a smaller number of hospitals which will be complemented by an increase in locally provided services. This multiplicity of 'hospitals' working in a networked interdependent system is summarised in Figure 1.6.

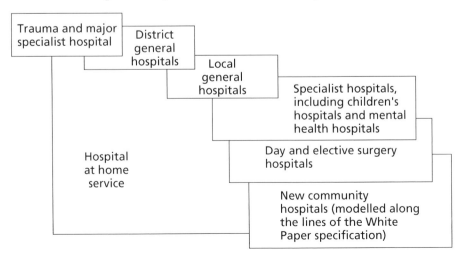

Figure 1.6 The 'hospital' network for local communities.

Developing the workforce

'Good Doctors, Safer Patients' – the regulation of doctors

The Chairman of the Shipman Inquiry, Dame Janet Smith, made serious criticisms of the current medical regulation system and the General Medical Council (GMC) and she made recommendations to update them with the objective of protecting patients and improving their safety.[30] The Chief Medical Officer (CMO) for England, working with the CMOs for Northern Ireland, Scotland and Wales, has undertaken a broad review and he has submitted detailed recommendations in a report: 'Good doctors, safer patients.' This report proposes measures to strengthen the arrangements for the protection of patients including devolving some of the powers of the GMC to local (employer) level, changing its structure and function, and creating a new framework for doctors' revalidation.[31]

Sir Donald Irvine, the former president of the GMC, highlighted the key issues[32] which are summarised in Box 1.1.

Box 1.1 Key issues for doctors' revalidation.

- Defining what a good doctor is and the standards of professional practice for achieving that.
- Embedding these standards into the medical registration and licensure, certification for specialist and general practice, medical education and doctors' contracts of employment.
- Standardising the entry to the profession through a new national examination for all doctors applying for registration with the GMC for the first time.
- Ensuring doctors are competent to practice on a continuing basis through revalidation embracing relicensure and recertification.
- Locating the regulation of doctors within the wider set of systems for improving and quality assuring modern practice.
- Establishing a more robust management and fairer process when there are concerns about a doctors' practice by placing greater emphasis on retraining and rehabilitation, having access to a workplace GMC affiliate and separating the investigation and adjudications in fitness to practice cases.
- Adopting a civil rather than a criminal standard of proof in fitness to practice cases.

The Royal Colleges and specialist societies are to take lead responsibility for delivering the key recertification element of revalidation for their members thus spearheading the development of a strong professional and competent workforce.[31,32] In addition, the proposal is to bring together and consolidate responsibility for both undergraduate and postgraduate medical education on the (to be renamed) Postgraduate Medical Education and Training Board (PMETB) thus creating a continuum of education across the UK.[33]

Fitness to practice – medical staff

To underpin these proposed major changes, NHS employers will have an important role in ensuring that their doctors' appraisal processes are sufficiently rigorous and consistent across the UK. The six key functions which might be expected in reviewing individual doctors and their practices include:

1   ensuring that practice is safe
2   ensuring that practice is of a good standard
3   taking opportunities to improve practice
4   reviewing performance in relation to service goals, objectives and targets
5   identifying and meeting professional development and training needs
6   checking that conduct is honest and ethical, and that the individual behaves with integrity.[31]

The current system of medical appraisal in the NHS varies from a 'cosy chat with a sympathetic colleague' to a more rigorous form of assessment. For the proposed new process of revalidation to be effective, the system needs to be upgraded. It will need to be based on a valid and reliable assessment of a doctor's everyday standard of practice so as to enable a judgement to be made about how good that doctor is, about the safety of their practice, and about the extent to which quality is embedded in their everyday work.[9] The issue of embedding the notion of 'fairness' in the appraisal process as directed by employment law will mean that NHS employers will have to place greater emphasis on providing all doctors with the necessary support in the form of retraining and 'rehabilitation'.

The regulation of the non-medical healthcare professions

In a parallel development, the Department of Health for England, working under the Government's reserve powers with colleagues in Northern Ireland, Scotland and Wales, has proposed a set of complementary reforms for the regulation of the non-medical healthcare professions.[34] The recommendations are summarised below:

• the regulation of the professions should form one integrated and consistent framework across the different professions, and should link up better with the measures employers take to satisfy themselves that their staff are working safely
• the creation of a more independent adjudication process about cases where someone's fitness to practice causes concern
• the need to provide objective and robust assurance that individual professionals remain fit to practice by standardising the content and enhancing the value of work place appraisal
• every registered professional will need to revalidate, but the amount of detail they need to provide will vary depending on how much risk to patients their work creates
• a major employer role in revalidation, with a system to check that employers fulfil this duty with parallel arrangements where there is no employer.

The proposals also include that the revalidation system should be both formative, an aid to development, and summative, a check that a required standard is met. Within the NHS, information gathered under the Knowledge and Skills Framework (KSF) should be the basis of revalidation. Within this context, the issue of identifying common educational standards such as the knowledge needed to underpin safe prescribing has been flagged for the attention of the regulators and the Council for Healthcare Regulatory Excellence.

Knowledge management and its developments

The concept of 'knowledge management' – the facilitation of the acquisition, sharing, storage, retrieval and utilisation of knowledge – is a relatively new field of study. Easterby-Smith and Lyles have distinguished several research domains which are summarised in Figure 1.7 and set within the two intersecting dichotomies of theory and practice, and process and content.[35]

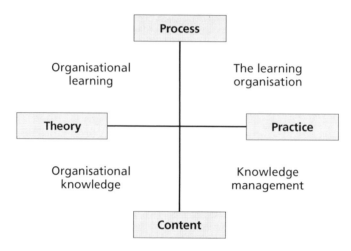

Figure 1.7 The knowledge management framework.

Given the proposed changes to the regulations and appraisal processes discussed above, the NHS will have to develop more robust approaches to supporting individual doctors' and professional staff's education and training needs through developing a knowledge management strategy for clinicians. Easterby-Smith and Lyles point out that knowledge management also has to sit within the context of the organisation's social architecture of knowledge exchange. This is potentially an important issue in the NHS and it has been embraced by the NHS major investment programme in clinical informatics and Information Technology (IT).[36]

To illustrate the depth of these developments for example, in England, two work streams are focusing on the national knowledge service and clinical practice and process; the key elements are shown in Table 1.3.

Table 1.3 The clinical knowledge management programme.

The national knowledge service	The clinical practice and process
• Best current knowledge service	• Better prescribing
• The national library for health	• Risk minimisation
• The nursing knowledge toolbox	• Clinician professional development
• National decision support service	• Do once and share
• The map of medicine	• The busy clinician
• NHS search engine	• National clinical toolbox
• Integrated child health knowledge	• The connected patient

The management agenda for AHPs

The Public Service Reform Agenda and the NHS multi-layered strategy for modernisation is extensive, complex and potentially difficult.

In concluding this chapter, the following watch list of key issues that AHP services managers, especially in England, might usefully focus on as they prioritise their work over the next two to three years is offered in Box 1.2.

Box 1.2 A watch list for AHP managers.

1 Work with the local commissioners as they try to define the programmes of care which therapists deliver even if the artificial boundaries seem inadequate as descriptions of your service.

2 Work with the tariff teams (in England) to establish the best level of accuracy for the cost of the programme as this affects your future budgets.

3 Work with your chief executive to rigorously control costs, especially on staff, and manage the cash flows for your service.

4 Work with your medical and nursing directors to build-up a sensible and robust approach to implementing the new regulations and the new quality assurance processes, liaising with the Health Professions Council and professional bodies as necessary.

5 Develop new practices and ways of working within the management context of maintaining rigorous financial controls and practice quality assurance.

6 Work with colleagues from the '3rd sector' in a collaborative network to ensure as best as you can, that the movement of the patients' care between agencies is a smooth as it can be.

7 Build-up a training, development and succession plan so as your senior staff start to retire, new members of staff can maintain the work you have set in train outlined above.

8 Stay up to date on the Government's policies and laws as they are being updated constantly.

9 Stay in touch with patients' and carers' opinions about your service and address their concerns.

10 Build-up a reputation for quality and excellence.

Author's note

It has been difficult to write this chapter as the Government's Public Policy Reform Agenda is too extensive to describe in detail here. However, it is critically important to have some familiarity with this agenda as it gives the context for understanding the National Health Service (NHS) policy direction.

Many thanks are due to our clients who have helped me to formulate my thinking over the years. In particular I would like to acknowledge the very helpful feedback I received from the senior officers of the NHS UK Medicines Information Service on a strategy paper I prepared for them in 2006. Their comments have helped me to clarify and improve my writing, and I believe their efforts will benefit AHP managers in this more sharply focused review of the Public Policy Reform Agenda and the NHS strategic direction.

References

1 Royal Commission on Long Term Care. *With Respect to Old Age: long term care – rights and responsibilities.* London: The Stationery Office; 1999.

2 Audit Commission. *The Coming of Age: improving care services for older people.* London: Audit Commission; 1997.

3 Audit Commission. *Forget Me Not: mental health services for older people.* London: Audit Commission; 1999.

4 Audit Commission. *Fully Equipped: the provision of equipment to older or disabled people by the NHS and social services in England and Wales.* London: Audit Commission; 2000.

5 Audit Commission. *Charging with Care: How Councils Charge for Home Care.* London: Audit Commission; 2000.

6 Audit Commission. *The Way to Go Home: rehabilitation and remedial services for older people.* London: Audit Commission; 2000.

7 Department of Health. *Improving Chronic Disease Management.* Available at: www.dh.gov.uk/organisation.

8 Department of Health. *The Expert Patient – a new approach to chronic disease management for the 21st century.* London: Department of Health; 2001.

9 Ham C, York N, Sutch S, *et al*. Hospital bed utilisation in the NHS, Kaiser Permanente, and the US Medicine programme: analysis of routine data. *BMJ.* 2003; **327**: 1257.

10 Department of Health. *Our health, Our care, Our say: a new direction for community services.* London: Department of Health; 2006.

11 Department for Education and Skills. *The Education and Inspections Act 2006.* Available at: www.dfes.gov.uk/publications/educationandinspectionsact/index.shtml.

12 Carter P. Managing Offenders, Reducing Crime – a new approach. *Correctional Services Review.* Home Office. 2003; 11 December.

13 Blunkett D. *Reducing crime – changing lives – the Government's plan for transforming the management of offenders.* Home Office. 2004; January.

14 www.probation.homeoffice.gov.uk/files/pdf/master%2020pp%20BB.pdf.

15 Department for Work and Pensions. *Pathways to Work: helping people into employment.* www.dwp/gov/uk/consultations/consult/2002/pathways/pathways.pdf.

16 DWP Press Release: 25th January 2005 www.dwp/gov/uk/consultations/consult/2002/pathways/pathways.pdf.

17 Model Standing orders. Available at: www.dh. gov.uk/PublicationsAndStatistics/Publications/PublicationsPolicyAndGuidance).

18 The Higgs Review. Available at: www.dti.gov.uk/bbf/corp-governance/higgs-tyson/page23342.html.

19 Arm's Length Bodies Review in the NHS and Social Care system for England. Available at: www.dh.gov.uk/AboutUs/DeliveringHealthAndSocialCare/OrganisationsThatWorkWithDH/ArmslengthBodies/fs/en.

20 Health Foundation. *A review of the Effectiveness of Primary Care-led Commissioning and Its Place in the NHS,* October 2004. Available at: http://www.health.org.uk/mediaroom/pressreleases/index.cfm?id=58forasummar

21 Secretary of State for Health. Patient Choice the key to NHS future. Speech given at the King's Fund, London, 14 June 2006. Available at: www.labour.org.uk/index.php?id=news

22 Payment by Results. Overview, Progress and Work Schedule Reports. Available at: www.dh.gov.uk/PolicyAndGuidance/OrganisationalPolicy/FinanceandPlanning/NHSFinancialReforms/fs/en.

23 Designed For Life. Available at: www.wales.nhs.uk/sites3/page.cfm?orgid= 452&pid= 11608).

24 Scottish Executive. *Health and Community Care Programme and NHS Health Scotland's Programme of Work.* Available at: http://www.scotland.gov.uk/topics/health and http://www.healthscotland.com.

25 Royal College of Surgeons of England and the British Orthopaedic Association's Report. *Better Care for the Severely Injured.* London: RCS; 2000.

26 Royal College of Surgeons of England. Reconfiguration Working Party Report. *Delivering High-quality Surgical Services for the Future.* London: RCS; 2006.

27 Royal College of Surgeons of England. National Collaborating Centre for Acute Care. *National Clinical Guidelines on Head Injury: triage, assessment, investigation and early management of head injuries in infants, children and adults.* London: RCS; 2003.

28 Royal College of Surgeons of England. *Professional Standards and Regulations: developing a modern surgical workforce.* London: RCS; 2005.

29 NHS Modernisation Agency hosted Critical Care Networks for the English Trusts' Networks and Contacts. Available at: www.modern.nhs.uk/scripts/default.asp?site id=20&id=7117.

30 The Shipman Inquiry. *Safeguarding Patients: lessons from the past, proposals for the future.* London: Stationary Office; 2004.

31 Department of Health.*Good doctors, safer patients: proposals to strengthen the system to assure and improve the performance of doctors and to protect the safety of patients.* DH: London; July 2006. Available at: www.dh.gov.uk/PublicationsAndStatistics/Publications.

32 Irvine D. Editorial. *Journal of the Royal Society of Medicine;* vol 99, September 2006. Available at: www.rsm.ac.uk/media/pr209.htm.

33 www.pmetb.org.uk.

34 Department of Health.*The regulation of the non-medical healthcare professions: a review by the Department of Health.* July 2006. Available at: www.dh.gov.uk/PublicationsAnd Statistics/Publications

35 Easterby-Smith M, Lyles MA. Watersheds of Organisational Learning and Knowledge Management. In: *Handbook of Organisational Learning and Knowledge Management.* Oxford: Blackwells; 2003.

36 Department for Health. Connecting for Health. Available at: www.connecting forhealth.nhs.uk/delivery/serviceimplementation/kps.

Further reading

- www.iod.com/intershoproot/ecs/store/en/pdfs/Higgsresponse.pdf.
- http://news.bbc.co.uk/l/hi/business/1780075.stm and 2096445.stm.
- http://specials.ft.com/enron.
- Wade E, Smith J, Peck E, *et al.* Health Service Management Centre review of PCT commissioning. In: *Commissioning in the reformed NHS: policy into practice.* University of Birmingham: Birmingham; March 2006.
- New Local Government Network think-tank piece – Making Choices: How Can Choice Improve Public Services? Available at: www.nlgn.org.uk.
- Labour Party Manifesto. Chapter 4. Section: Empowering patients: choosing not waiting. 2005. Available at: www.labour.org.uk/fileadmin/manifesto.
- The 'Bedfordshire' Ruling on a patient's choice. Available at: http:// news.bbc.co.uk/1/hi/england/beds/bucks/herts/3156838.stm.
- Welsh Assembly Government. Health Minister Dr. Brian Gibbons's interview with BBC Wales News – 19.5.2005. Available at: http://news.bbc.co.uk/1/hi/wales/4560653.stm.
- The Healthcare Commission Report. Acute hospital portfolio – Accident and Emergency. 2004. Available at: www.healthcarecommission.org.uk/serviceproviderinformation/ reviews&inspections.
- The Department of Health. Report on Modernising Emergency Care and the Ambulance Service. June 2006. Available at: www.dh.gov.uk/AdvancedSearch.
- The infrastructure of evidence-based performance metrics developed for cardiac surgeons by the Society for Cardiothoracic Surgery in Great Britain and Ireland and the Healthcare Commission. Available at: http://heartsurgery.healthcarecommission.org.uk.

Chapter 2

Managing change: a Framework for the Management of Change

Robert Jones and Fiona Jenkins

Everything flows and nothing stays
You can't step twice into the same river[1]

Introduction

Change is an every day occurrence for all healthcare staff whether managers, clinicians or members of support teams. The way in which change is embraced and managed impacts on the care provided for patients as well as the success of organisations, services and personal job satisfaction. As managers of healthcare services it is imperative that we have an understanding of the theoretical concepts of change management and the practical skills to lead and manage change. Our aim in this chapter is to provide an overview and insight into this important sphere of management, to introduce and focus on our 'Framework for the Management of Change' and to set out some case studies which are examples of successful change management projects based on the 'Framework' and from our own experience as managers and leaders in the AHPs and wider healthcare. The chapter also relates closely to the next chapter in this volume which is focused on the development of care pathways incorporating many elements of change management and leadership.

Throughout the last hundred years academics and practitioners have developed a very extensive body of literature on the theory and practice of change management including the development of a wide range of concepts, models, tools and techniques – there are many schools of thought with an ever increasing literature supporting the evidence-base. For this reason, it has not been possible here to set out a detailed analysis of this vast and complex field of theory and practice, but to provide a selective review and positive guidance.

Change

Everyone finds change difficult: according to Samuel Johnson,[2] 'Change is not made without inconvenience, even from worse to better,' and it is clear from the literature on the management and leadership of change that there is no 'right' 'best' or only one way of doing it. Bernard Burnes [3] recognises that:

What almost everyone would like is a clear and practical change theory which explains what changes organisations need to make and how they should make them. Unfortunately, what is available is a wide range of confusing and contradictory theories, approaches and recipes. Many of these are well thought out and grounded in both theory and practice; others, unfortunately, seem disconnected from either theory or reality. Also, though change theory requires an interdisciplinary perspective, each of the major approaches tends to view organisations from the disciplinary angles of their originators – whether it be psychology, sociology, economics, or whatever – which can result in an incomplete and biased picture. So, regardless of what their proponents may claim, we do not possess at present an approach to change that is theoretically holistic, universally applicable, and which can be practically applied.

Change management is not a distinct discipline with rigid and clearly defined boundaries, but rather the theory and practice draws on a wide range of social science disciplines and traditions. Something that is certain is that all of us – whoever we are and whatever we do – are involved in, subject to and bringers about of change in the working environment whatever our roles, grades or professions.

Change is one of the few constants of recorded history.[1, 2]

Often society's 'winners', both historical and contemporary, can be characterised by their common ability to effectively manage and exploit change situations … Management and change are synonymous, it is impossible to undertake a journey – for in many respects that is what change is – without first addressing the purpose of the trip, the route you wish to travel and with whom.[4]

In Chapter 1 of this book, Patricia Oakley sets out, explores and examines the Government work programme for 2006–07 to 2009–10 of public policy reforms and the NHS strategic development agenda. There are many elements which make up the 'jigsaw of reform' with very significant implications for AHPs and all other NHS managers and staff, including for example:

- developing service commissioning and accountability
- performance management
- reducing risk
- maintaining financial control
- developing service providers – including the 'third sector'
- developing the workforce
- the changing legal and regulatory framework.

It is clear from these examples that the pace and intensity of change will continue unabated and will continue to affect all those working in healthcare; it is therefore essential that managers and staff from all backgrounds develop strategies for proactively managing and leading, handling and participating in change processes.

Change management can be approached from a variety of different angles and applied to numerous organisational processes. To be effective, it needs to be multi-disciplinary, touching all aspects of the organisation. An essential element in implementing new procedures, technologies, ways of working and so on and overcoming resistance to change is through effective involvement of all. A complex interplay of emotions and cognitive processes bear on attitudes to change; people therefore react to change differently. On the positive side, change may be seen as opportunity, renewal, rejuvenation, progress, innovation or growth whilst on the other hand – and equally legitimately – it might be seen as upheaval, instability, threat, disorientation and unpredictability. Whether change is perceived as frightening, demoralising or the source of anxiety and stress or approached with excitement, enthusiasm and confidence, or somewhere between these, is dependent on many factors including the psychological make up of individuals, the actions of managers and leaders, the behaviour and ethos of the organisation or service and the nature, scope and impact of the proposed change. People facing change may experience a whole series of negative emotions such as anger, denial, frustration or simply acceptance and resignation. All of these feelings need to be overcome when working toward committed and enthusiastic change implementation. In order to create change in a positive and lasting way, these perceptions cannot be ignored however difficult they may be. An important aspect of change management must be to involve staff at all levels including everyone in defining the nature of the change required and the subsequent processes, not simply imposing change.

Key concepts

There is an extensive and complex literature on the management and leadership of change and the challenges it produces.[3, 4, 5, 6, 7, 8, 9, 10, 11] In Chapter 7 of the first book in this series, *Managing and Leading in the Allied Health Professions*,[12] Christina Pond also provides a detailed analysis and discussion of leadership which is an important adjunct to this and our next chapter in this volume on care pathways.

NHS management and organisational structures have been the subject of radical and constant change since the 1974 structural reorganisation[13] and the pace of 'reform' now seems to increase on an almost daily basis. Hooper and Potter[14] suggest that there are 'five key drivers' for change which, when combined with accurate timing – implementing change before a peak in performance is reached – which allows latent energy from the previous change cycle to be used while still at the experimental stage of the new cycle. Hooper and Potter[8] stress the importance of leadership in maintaining the momentum of change linking this with the 'sigmoid curve' – shown in Figure 2.1 – originally expounded by Charles Handy.[6] The

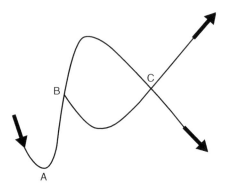

Figure 2.1 Learning dip and sigmoid curve.

sigmoid – 'S' shaped curve represents the life cycle of an individual or an organisation which always waxes and then wanes. When starting a change project, there is an initial 'learning dip' before progress is quickly made. It is important to start the second curve at point 'A' before the peak, harnessing the 'latent energy' of experience from the old curve while still at the experimental stage.

Burnes[15] cites three schools of thought:

1 **the individual perspective school**: supporters of this theory include the behaviourists who believe that behaviour results from an individual's interaction with their environment and the Gestalt-Field psychologists, who argue that an individual's behaviour is the product of behaviour and reason
2 **the group dynamic school**: this school has the longest history; its emphasis is about bringing organisational change through teams or work groups rather than individuals. The rationale is that because organisations work in groups, individual behaviour must be seen, modified or changed in the light of groups' prevailing practices/postulating that group behaviour is an intricate set of symbolic interactions and forces which affect group structure and modify individual behaviours. The group brings about tensions that put pressures on its members
3 **the open systems school**: the primary reference for this school is the organisation in its entirety. It suggests that any change to one part of the organisation will have an impact on all the other parts due to interconnected sub-systems and in turn an effect on performance. However the organisation is not seen in isolation and is open to – and interacts with – the external environment as well as being open internally to the other sub-systems in the organisation. The objective of this approach is to structure the functions of the business in a manner that clearly defines lines of co-ordination and interdependence emphasising achieving synergy rather than optimising performance of any one individual part.

In their discussion of the importance of managing change and how to handle the resultant anxiety that is associated with change, Obholzer and Roberts[16] emphasise the importance of understanding the different aspects of anxiety and its origins. Baker and Perkins[17] in their study of healthcare practitioners commented that change needs to be planned and managed, since the effective operation of a complex service is dependent on the goodwill, competence and co-operation of its staff – change, they assert, can also threaten the efficiency of an organisation.

Pettigrew, Ferlie and McKee[18] in their study of a variety of NHS changes proposed the concept of 'receptive' and 'non-receptive' contexts for change. Schon[19] argued that there is a 'conservative dynamic' within most organisations that strives to resist change; the positive side of this being the stability that is provided during times when change is not taking place.

Successful change according to Lewin[20] requires the 'unfreezing' of current attitudes, systems and behaviours. He proposed that a programme of planned change and improved performance incorporates a three-phase process:

1 *unfreezing* – reducing the forces that maintain the status quo; recognising the need for change and improvement to take place
2 *transition* – the development of new attitudes or behaviours and implementation of the change
3 *refreezing* – stabilising the change at the new level and supporting mechanisms in place to reinforce the change.

Burnes[3] set out a further range of change initiatives including Total Quality Management (TQM) and Business Process Re-engineering (BPR). He concluded that change programmes were not guaranteed to succeed, but that the theory and practice of change management were an 'essential requisite for survival'.

Culture

A study of the concepts of attitudes and behaviours linked to management within an organisation introduces the concept of 'culture'. Schein[21] suggests that culture evolves as a complex outcome of external pressure, internal potential, critical events and chance and proposed that cultural understanding is essential for leaders. Organisational culture – an important aspect which is often overlooked – warrants attention in change management processes. He proposed that culture and leadership are two sides of the same coin and could not be understood on their own; suggesting that the only thing of real importance that leaders do is to create and manage culture. Also he asserts that culture is in a sense a learned product of group experience and is to be found only when there is a definable group with a significant history. Therefore, according to Schein, a new group would have had no culture at the beginning, as it had no history. He suggests that culture evolves as a complex outcome of external pressures, internal potential, critical events and chance.

Handy[22] had a different perspective suggesting the four dominant cultures of:

1 club
2 role
3 task
4 person.

Schneider and Barsoux[23] discuss the interdependency between culture and structure. They commented on the different management styles adopted in Latin managers – who like formal structures and power division. Whereas cultural styles and power division cultural styles are adopted by Nordic and Anglo managers – who believe that the world is too complex to be able to clearly define roles and functions. They concluded that effectively transferring management structures and processes rely on the ability to recognise inherent assumptions and compare with cultural assumptions.

The NHS has many cultures including; an overall public sector culture, sub-cultures at individual organisational level, profession or occupational group sub-cultures and team. The importance of 'identity' and 'belonging' need to be acknowledged when introducing management reorganisation as lack of awareness of the importance of culture may be detrimental to the success of change management. Cultural changes take longer to accomplish than organisational restructuring, but an understanding of culture will help to facilitate effective change programmes.

Leadership

A clear understanding of leadership skills and techniques is essential for the success of any change management project.[12] The role and personality of a leader may be seen as the critical determinant of change management. Kotter[24] estimated that successful leadership – rather than management – is responsible for a high percentage of successful change. Handy[7] also suggests that leadership theory falls into categories of:

- trait
- style
- contingency.

Bennis and Nannus[10] have suggested that leadership has three main aspects:

1 commitment
2 complexity
3 credibility.

Leadership vision was discussed by Wesley and Mintzberg[25] who proposed that most authors agree with the assertion that leadership vision can be broken into three stages of: envisioning, communicating effectively with followers, and empowering. Hooper and Potter,[14] draw together concepts of Transactional, Transformational and Transcendent leadership, detailing the change from command and control leadership, through to empowerment. This theory has developed changes and evolution in leadership style.

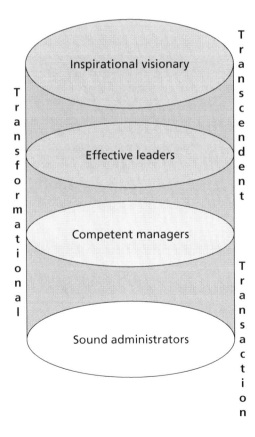

Figure 2.2 A hierarchy of leadership.

Potter describes three levels of leadership: team, operational and strategic[26] other authors also suggest that leadership concepts are sub-divided into three levels using a variety of terminologies, there is a degree of consensus surrounding many of the theories of leadership introducing the human relations aspect of change.

The concept of emotional intelligence was introduced by Daniel Goleman[12,27,28] describing this as the ability to manage ourselves and our relationships effectively, with the four fundamental capabilities of:

1 self-awareness
2 self-management
3 social awareness
4 social skill.

Mastery of these areas, he argued, could enable the leader to choose the leadership style required for any given situation including when undertaking change management.

Teams

There are many theories relating to team working. The difference between teams that perform well and others that do not, is a subject that is often accorded too little attention in the context of management and leadership of change. Part of the problem might be that 'team' is a word and concept familiar to everyone in a wide range of contexts.

Team working and leadership are discussed in detail by Katzenback and Smith[29] who emphasise the need for 'team purposing' when working collectively. They suggest that teams and good performance are inextricably linked. Their research shows that it is basic discipline that enables teams to work. Teams and good performance are inseparable, they argue; you can't have one without the other. Teamwork encompasses a set of values that encourage listening and responding constructively to views expressed by others.

> However, good performance can be attributed to other factors. There is a distinct difference between a group of people brought together as a 'team', and a group that has a common vision and purpose. The latter produces individual efforts and 'collective work products' i.e. more than the sum of the individual contributors. The core is common commitment; which is only seen by a purposing team.[29]

Hirshhorn[30] highlights the damaging effect of interpersonal conflict that can occur within teams, making them dysfunctional.

Models, techniques and approaches for change management

The management and leadership of change is both an imprecise science and art. However, there is a large, extensive evidence-base from which to draw, including a wide range of theories and models – old and new – which might be applied to differing circumstances.

Before moving on to present our own 'Framework for the Management of Change' a brief overview of a few examples of the possible models, techniques and approaches in this complex area may be useful to refer to. However, this review is far from exhaustive as Figure 2.3 adapted from Iles and Sutherland[5] – which lists some examples – shows. It is intended to be useful to facilitate further exploration and for reference:

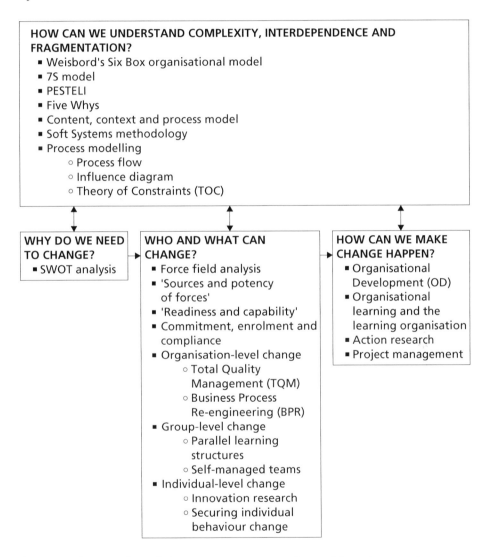

HOW CAN WE UNDERSTAND COMPLEXITY, INTERDEPENDENCE AND FRAGMENTATION?
- Weisbord's Six Box organisational model
- 7S model
- PESTELI
- Five Whys
- Content, context and process model
- Soft Systems methodology
- Process modelling
  - Process flow
  - Influence diagram
  - Theory of Constraints (TOC)

WHY DO WE NEED TO CHANGE?
- SWOT analysis

WHO AND WHAT CAN CHANGE?
- Force field analysis
- 'Sources and potency of forces'
- 'Readiness and capability'
- Commitment, enrolment and compliance
- Organisation-level change
  - Total Quality Management (TQM)
  - Business Process Re-engineering (BPR)
- Group-level change
  - Parallel learning structures
  - Self-managed teams
- Individual-level change
  - Innovation research
  - Securing individual behaviour change

HOW CAN WE MAKE CHANGE HAPPEN?
- Organisational Development (OD)
- Organisational learning and the learning organisation
- Action research
- Project management

Figure 2.3 An overview of change management tools, models and approaches.

We set out below a selection of examples of various approaches which might be helpful in a variety of change management circumstances. These outlines are not intended as a 'how to do it' guide but as an indication of the range of models methodologies and techniques available.

Change process steps. Bristow *et al* [31] outlined a process through which change development could be achieved.

> **Box 2.1 Processes for development.**
>
> - Recognise need for change
> - Seek help as required
> - Diagnose problem
> - Decide direction of change
> - Develop change plan
> - Evaluate and review
> - Continue cycle of development.

Seven phases to social change intervention using an external 'Change Agent'. In this example an external 'change agent' is brought into the organisation to facilitate the change process.[32] The 'client' is the 'host' organisation. Generally change programmes are managed internally within the organisation without input from external sources.

Table 2.1 Seven phases to social change intervention.

Phase	Action
1 Develop the need for change	Begin unfreezing with problem awareness on the part of one or more managers/leaders
2 Establish the change relationship	Preliminary exploration between 'change agent' and client
3 Diagnose the planned system's problem	Collaborative data collection and analysis between change agent and client system
4 Examine alternatives and action goals	Stage change by determining action strategies and plans
5 Implement actions	Change activities and obtain feedback about results
6 Generalise and stabilise the change	Provide reinforcement to ensure workable changes are retained without backsliding
7 Evaluate and terminate 'Change Agent' relationship	Develop mechanisms for ongoing internal adjustment

8-Stage process of change. Wesley and Mintzberg[25] proposed an '8-stage' process of change.

> **Box 2.2 8-Stage process of change.**
>
> 1 Establishing a sense of urgency.
> 2 Creating the guiding coalition.
> 3 Developing vision and strategy.
> 4 Communicating the change vision.
> 5 Empowering employees for broad-based action.
> 6 Generating short-term 'wins'.
> 7 Consolidating gains and producing more change.
> 8 Anchoring new approaches in the culture.

Change curve – reactions to change. The 'Change Curve' (Figure 2.4) represents the personal transitions and emotions a person tends to go through as they work through the change process. The reactions and responses generally follow a particular pattern. The challenges for managers are to get the systems, process and structures right and also, importantly, to help and support staff through the change process.

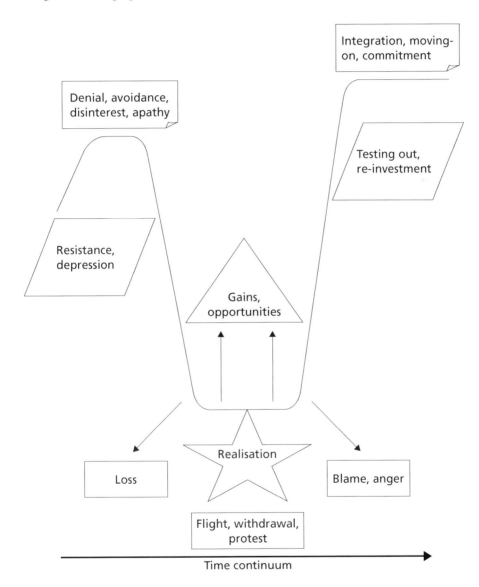

Figure 2.4 Reactions to change.

Iceberg process. The flow of tasks involved in implementing change is very often impeded by the underlying, submerged issues and behaviours. The barriers or resistance may have little to do with the rationale of the task being undertaken and everything to do with the feelings and relationships surrounding the task.

Therefore, awareness of the process is in itself not enough, process has to be consciously managed and lead.

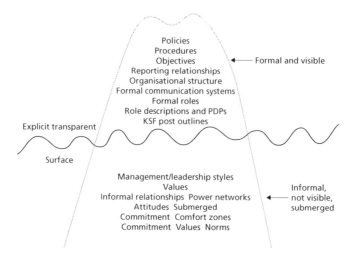

Figure 2.5 Iceberg process.

Force field analysis. The diagnostic technique of 'Force Field Analysis' is used as a method of looking at variables involved in determining whether change will occur. It is based on the idea of 'forces' relating to perceptions about particular factors and their influences. Driving forces are those which 'push' in a particular direction, initiating change or keeping it going while restraining forces are acting to decrease the driving force or restraining it. It is a dynamic system approach to change and sees all situations as temporary and potentially changeable. At any given moment a field of forces are acting on an event or problem. The approach involves identifying the forces and seeking to change their direction or strength.

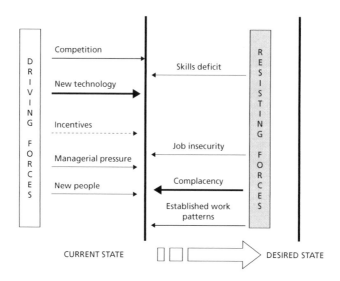

Figure 2.6 Force field analysis.

PDSA analysis. During the 1930s the PDSA cycle was developed as a model for process improvement in the context of change. It has been used ever since and was much vaunted by the NHS Modernisation Agency and is widely used as one of the techniques available in the management and leadership of change processes. The model illustrates the four phases of the PDSA cycle – Plan, Do, Study, Act – that may be used as part of improving a process or processes.

The phases of the PDSA cycle are:

- **P**lan what you are going to do after gathering evidence of the nature and size of the problem
- **D**o it, preferably on a small scale first
- **S**tudy the results to ascertain whether a plan works
- **A**ct on the results, if the plan was successful standardise on the new way of working, if not successful, try an alternative.

See also Chapter 3 of this volume on development of care pathways.

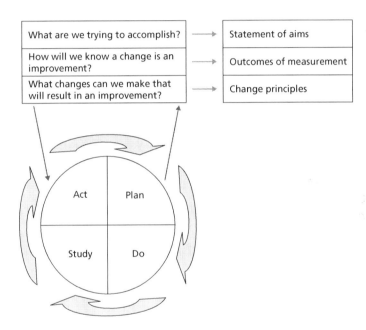

Figure 2.7 PDSA cycle.

SWOT analysis

Subject of S.W.O.T. Analysis here; define the subject of the analysis here

Strengths
Advantages of proposition
Workforce
Capabilities
Competitive advantages
Unique selling points
Resources, assets
Experience, knowledge, data
Financial reserves likely returns
Marketing–reach, distribution,
    awareness
Innovative aspects
Location and geographical
Price, value, quality
Accreditations, qualifications
Processes, systems, IT,
    communications
Cultural, attitudinal, behavioural
Management and succession

Weaknesses
Disadvantages of proposition
Gaps in capabilities
Lack of competitive strength
Reputation, presence and reach
Financial
Known vulnerabilities
Timescales, deadlines and
    pressures
Cost
Continuity
Effects on core activities,
    distraction
Reliability of data, plan
    predictability
Morale, commitment, leadership
Accreditations
Processes and systems
Management issues and succession

Opportunities
Market development
Competitors' vulnerabilities
Lifestyle trends
Technology development,
    innovation
Wider influences
New markets–vertical, horizontal
Niche target markets
Geographical
New unique selling points
Business developments
Information and research
Partnerships
Volumes, economies

Threats
Political effects
Legislative effects
Environmental effects
IT developments
Competitor intentions
Market demand
New technologies, services, ideas
Vital contracts and partners
Sustaining internal capabilities
Obstacles faced
Insurmountable weaknesses
Loss of key staff
Sustainable financial backing
Resistance to change
Home economy

Figure 2.8 SWOT analysis.

PEST analysis

```
Insert subject for P.E.S.T. analysis–business, proposition...
```

Political
Environmental issues
Current legislation
Future legislation
European/international legislation
Regulatory bodies and processes
Government policies
Government term and change
Funding, grants and initiatives
Home and international lobbying/
    pressure groups

Economic
Economic situation and trends
Market trends
Customer/end-user drivers

Social
Lifestyle trends
Demographics
Consumer attitudes and opinions
Media views
Law changes affecting social factors
Brand, technology image
Major events and influences
Role models
Access
Ethnic/religious factors
Advertising and publicity
Ethical issues

Technological
Competing technology development
Research funding
Associated/dependent technologies
Replacement technology/solutions
Maturity of technology
Capacity
Information and communications
Technology legislations
Innovation potential

Figure 2.9 PEST analysis.

Communicating change

Change programmes sometimes fail and should not rely on 'Big Bang' announcements to persuade staff to 'fall in line'; this method is never advisable, leading to unsustainable change. Existing communication channels may be inadequate to report progress, particularly with a substantial change programme. When staff do not receive the information they need they may turn to the 'grape vine' the challenge for managers is to ensure that communication is timely, accurate and all inclusive.

Saunders[33] reports a study that shows:

- 20% of an organisation's employees tend to support change from the outset
- 50% are 'fence sitters'
- 30% are 'resistors' whom nothing can sway.

Communication strategy should therefore be initially aimed at the 70% supporters and 'fence sitters'.

Box 2.3 Communication strategy.

1 Be specific about the change – staff should see the change programme as a tangible goal at organisational or departmental level, for example, reduce length of stay by three days.

2 Explain – to avoid staff feeling left in the dark about the reasons why change is required. Managers may have studied in depth the reasons why, but these need communicating to staff.

3 Let staff know the scope of the change – even when the news is not good. Rumours can be worse than reality, it is better to inform staff if changes to staff numbers or redundancies are needed.

4 Ensure two-way communication – meeting with staff to listen to their views as well as to inform is vital to offer explanation but also to gather ideas from the 'front line'.

5 Be repetitive about the change plans and actions – if staff hear the message several times they will be clear about the message, the reasons for change and the consequences of not addressing the problem.

6 Use pictures and graphs – many people retain information best if they see it visually.

7 Use multiple methods for communication – posters, flyers, emails, letters, videos in staff canteens, web based information as well as the invaluable one-to-one or group meetings are all avenues to be explored to get key messages across to staff and stakeholders.

8 Gain middle manager support – use this tier of management effectively they are key to implementing the programme and have significant influence in the organisation.

9 Offer training – training to build up new skills will support staff who need to be confident that the new system will work, equipped with new skills they will support the process.

10 Model the changes yourself – it is important that managers embrace the change themselves – rather than just expect staff to change – words and actions need to be consistent with the change strategy.

Change leadership

Managers need to develop a range of leadership competencies to ensure the success of change programmes.

How to overcome 'change fatigue'

All organisational change involves three phases:[34]

1 initial recognition and preparation; design of a response to set goals
2 implementation of changes; the period of often 'hard won' change
3 consolidation period; when the organisation reviews and adjusts.

The three phases are not linear and the second one is often considered to be the most difficult where resistors need to be brought 'on board'. Change programmes may fail for two main reasons:

Table 2.2 Change leadership.

	Organisational change agenda	Leadership competency profile
Creating value	• Customer focus	• Focus on client value Cultivate relationships
	• Innovate and be creative	• Drive innovation
	• Outcome focus	• Deliver results consistently
Executing strategy	• Mission, vision, values	• Strategy shaping
	• Creativity and alignment Communicate openly	• Building commitment
	• Team work	• Team building and development
	• Sustainable change	• Develop organisational learning

1 poor design – where underlying processes, for example, the way resources are allocated, or waiting for the ideal IT solution and not addressing specific behavioural problems
2 poor communication – change leaders must be prepared to communicate the same message at least six times – to ensure the message is heard by all. Staff must hear the arguments for and against the change options; they also need to hear that the organisation will support them through the change process.

The change leader should avoid trying to detail in advance the precise shape of the future – as failure to reach this precision can be virtually guaranteed and this can be demoralising. A better tactic is to outline the goals at the outset and improvise as the change project develops.

The key to substantive improvement lies in creating an environment in which change becomes part of the culture being continual, gradual and low level. Change is more effective and sustainable if it relies on staff motivation rather than directives downwards from the top of the organisation.

Critical mistakes and errors

In his article 'Why Transformation Efforts Fail', Kotter[35] identifies eight possible 'critical mistakes … errors' and why 'hard-won' gains may be negated:

Table 2.3 Leading change – why transformation efforts fail.

Error 1	Not establishing a great enough sense of urgency
Error 2	Not creating a powerful enough guiding coalition
Error 3	Lacking a vision
Error 4	Under communicating the vision by a factor of ten
Error 5	Not removing obstacles to the new vision
Error 6	Not systematically planning for and creating short-term wins
Error 7	Declaring victory too soon
Error 8	Not anchoring changes in the organisations culture

Key factors in effective change management

Paton and McCalman[4] identified ten key factors in effective change management based on:

- innovative responses to triggers for change
- holistic solutions
- visionary leadership
- committed support.

The ten factors – they argue – must be addressed and actioned if:

> change is to be effectively managed. By ensuring that these factors have been considered before initiating change, the 'problem owner' and associated change agents will be in a position to confidently manage the process of transition…

A summary of the ten factors is shown in Table 2.4.

Table 2.4 Change management factors.

1 Change is all pervasive	Any change process is likely to have an impact greater than the sum of its parts. 'A holistic view must be taken to ensure that the full impact is understood'; look at the whole picture.
2 Effective change needs active senior management support	It is vital that senior managers support the change process.
3 Change is a multi-disciplinary activity	Most successful changes are brought about through team working. No one person is a 'change island', recognition of the multi-disciplinary nature of change is important in the sequence of achieving transformation.
4 Change is about people	People are the most important assets within an organisation or service; the team must be involved in the process from the outset, active participation is vital to gain commitment and 'ownership' of the change process. Change management is about people management and leadership. Essential elements are: • openness • good communication • involvement.
5 Change is about success	Dinosaur organisations and services become extinct through failure to adapt to the changing environment – it is important to set goals for success that can be achieved and be seen to be deliverable.
6 Change is a perpetual process	Something else always comes along to further impact: 'How do we explain change that was successful? How do we

explain change that never seemed to get going? How can we explain the change project that started off well, but seemed to fade away after a couple of years? The answers seem to lie in the attention and resources devoted to managing change as a perpetual process ... change is about identifying triggers, seeking vision, recruiting converts to the vision and maintaining and renewing the need for change management action is necessary on all these fronts'.[4]

7 Effective change requires competent change agents	Change agents (managers, leaders and teams) require appropriate skills, knowledge and position; a wide range of competencies are necessary for the achievement of successful outcomes. 'People skills' are essential and often difficult competencies to acquire.
8 There is no one best way or methodology	It is important not to take a 'blinkered' or 'singular' approach; what works for one change situation may not be appropriate to another.
9 Change is about 'ownership'	It is important that all involved feel 'ownership' and that the process is 'owned' by the problem owners, the change agents – managers, leaders and teams – and those affected by the change. It is also essential that the management team feel that they are responsible for the successful implementation of the change. This implies the concept of the management team moving from control to commitment and support. When people are coerced or manoeuvred into change situations by threat or crisis, the result is at best indifference and at worst resistance. When people 'own' the change process and feel that it offers opportunities they are much more likely to be committed to achieving a successful outcome.
10 Change is about fun, challenge and opportunity	'When faced with a challenge, most individuals respond positively. 'We use "fun", in this instance, to denote an attitude of mind ... throughout the seriousness of it all – the drive for performance, the need to maintain competitive edge, the desire for better, more effective organisation – there is also a need to show a human face'.[4]

Key behaviours and success factors

We have shown that there are many possible approaches, models, techniques and methodologies for bringing about successful change and there are no 'one only solutions' for moving from the current to a newly desired situation. However, we believe that there are a number of key behaviours and success factors that can usefully be identified to help make the process positive and which we have incorporated into our 'Framework for the Management of Change', including for example:

Table 2.5 Key behaviours and success factors.

Behaviours	Success factors
Pro-activity	A long term perspective
Inclusiveness, people involvement at all levels and across the whole team	Striving to achieve short- as well as long-term 'wins'
Flexibility	Development of vision and goals
Innovation	Using measures of success
Learning organisation/service	Benchmarking
Maintain focus	Maintain focus
Ability to use a variety of management styles	Use of appropriate knowledge and skills from within the team
Maintain calmness in challenging situation	Understanding the context
Integrity	Strategic level support
Honesty	Management support
Openness	Keep it simple at all times, over complexity loses time and context
Coaching	Manage and lead with a clearly defined and explicit set of organisational/service values
Excellent communication	Identification and implementation of appropriate training/education
Celebration of success	Celebration of success

These suggestions are not in specific priority order and are not all-inclusive.

Framework for the Management of Change

An essential part of every manager's work is the management of change. There are a multitude of different approaches and methods that can be taken to facilitate successful outcomes. We have developed a 'Framework for the Management of Change' that builds on theoretical evidence, combining this with our practical experience in this field of management. The framework is not proposed as a 'one only way of doing it' or 'recipe', but rather a template which indicates the necessary consideration and steps to be taken at each phase of the change process. The framework has been tested in a number of situations and has been shown to facilitate successful and sustainable service improvement.

   We developed the framework collaboratively with a view to facilitating specific change management projects. We wanted to incorporate established theory and practice into a simple methodology which could be adopted in a wide range of change situations and also support others in managing and leading change management processes.

Box 2.4 Framework for the Management of Change.

1 Moving from the current to the desired situation
- Identify 'triggers' for change
- Managerial imperatives
- Establish project group
- Shared vision, objectives and critical success factors

2 Essential actions
- Data and information
- Timing
- Setting the direction
- Staff participation at all levels
- Negotiation with stakeholders
- Specification phase
- Implementation
- Determine evaluation parameters

3 Skills for success
- Management:
  - i   responsibility, accountability, authority
  - ii   commitment
  - iii strategic thinking
  - iv   creativity
  - v   negotiating and influencing skills
  - vi   resources
  - vii political awareness
  - viii team working.
- Leadership:
  - i   clear vision and focus
  - ii   enthusiasm and commitment
  - iii communication
  - iv   ability to challenge 'comfort zones'
  - v   empowerment of staff at all levels
  - vi   ownership
  - vii create alignment.

4 Evaluation
- Completion within time-scale
- Completion within resources
- Success criteria
- Training
- Service user feedback
- Staff feedback
- Stakeholder feedback
- Adjust and re-evaluate

5 Learning points
- Understanding the context
- Constraints and barriers
- Clear vision of desired situation
- Importance of people
- Variety of management styles
- Communication – timely, frequent, open
- Infrastructure – organisational support
- Resilience

Case study 1 'Choice appointments'

'Choice appointments' an innovative appointment system for out-patient physiotherapy services.

In the autumn of 2003 an innovative system for out-patient physiotherapy appointments was introduced at Eastbourne District General Hospital. This service re-design initiative was intended to improve patient choice and control over the intervention and treatment programmes, decrease 'did not attends' (DNAs) and 'unable to attends', decrease waiting times, decrease the number of complaints about long waiting times and maximise clinical outcomes.

The system – designed in accord with our Framework for the Management of Change – enables routine physiotherapy musculo-skeletal out-patient referrals to book same-day appointments at times of their choice for both first appointments and follow-ups.

Moving from the current to the desired situation

• **Triggers for change**
Musculo-skeletal problems represent around 30% of all GP consultations and account for between 30% and 35% of physiotherapy services. Referral sources include GPs, consultants and their teams, self referral, and a range of other disciplines and professions.

The triggers for change included the volume of DNAs which on the departmental audit figures for the previous three years indicated a level of 11.3% per annum, significant wasted resources. Waiting times for non-urgent referrals were around fourteen weeks and there were several complaints per month relating to long waiting times for out-patient physiotherapy. There was a desire to offer patients more choice about the days and times of their attendance and give more control over the quantity of intervention to patients. A further assumption was that clinical outcomes would be further improved if interventions were quicker, rather than patients having to wait up to 14 weeks for first appointments – prompt intervention is clinically effective and patients want to get back to full function as quickly as possible.

• **Managerial imperatives**
To re-design the out-patient appointment system with the objective of eliminating DNAs, cutting waiting times, decreasing complaints about waiting times, improving patient control and choice, at no extra cost and striving to provide a responsive service for referrers and to be well within the requirements of commissioners.

These objectives were also in line with the political imperatives of providing greater choice for service users, cutting waste, contributing to the speed of throughput to support Trust waiting list initiatives and ensuring a responsive appointment booking system was in place – being 'in tune' with wider political agendas. It was also seen as important for the service to be 'well-positioned' for new developments being introduced into the NHS such as Payment by Results, Practice based Commissioning, Choose and Book and so on.

• **Establish project group**
The project group for this work was already in place; the group comprised the out-patients physiotherapy team led by the out-patient physiotherapy manager –

the team already met on a weekly basis and was augmented on an ad hoc basis as necessary to include other key staff such as the receptionist.

- **Shared vision, objectives and critical success factors**

Development of shared vision evolved over several meetings. The new system was unique and therefore had no template on which to build, or experience on which to draw. The overall aim was to introduce a system by which patients could book first appointments and follow-ups by phone on the days and for the times they wished to attend, basing the system on a capacity planning methodology. The key objectives were to: decrease DNAs, decrease waiting times, decrease complaints – improve patient satisfaction – offer greater choice and control to patients, ensure 'best quality possible' clinical outcomes, meet managerial and political imperatives. The critical success factors would comprise these aims and objectives which would be used as audit parameters to assess the success, or otherwise, of the system.

Essential actions

- **Data and information**

Timely, accurate and relevant data is required before the change process commences, as a background to underpin the development process. A wide range of data is required at all stages to facilitate management of the change project in all its aspects. Data collection, analysis and interpretation are crucial to all management work and wherever possible this should be supported by appropriate computerised information systems. Meaningful information can then be shared within the team and outside it, to facilitate the change management process.

- **Timing**

Time-scales were agreed within the team for implementation of the phases of development.

- **Setting the direction**

The direction of the project was led by the out-patient physiotherapy manager who also oversaw the development of paperwork and IM&T systems support. The physiotherapy manager was given responsibility for liaising with GPs, consultants and their teams and other interested parties.

- **Staff participation at all levels**

All members of the physiotherapy out-patient team were included at all stages of the development including reception staff, assistants, physiotherapists at all grades, clerical staff, the therapy services IM&T officer; patients and referrer's views were sought and represented by the out-patient physiotherapy manager. The head of therapy services supported the group and also acted as a liaison within the trust and outside.

- **Negotiation with stakeholders**

Stakeholders were involved and informed by the physiotherapy manager and head of therapy services. A number of specific negotiations also took place throughout the course of the development, for example, with a telephone company for the provision of a phone system at favourable terms. Commissioners were also kept fully informed of the development.

- **Specification phase**

The existing service had been fully reviewed in terms of measurement of DNAs, waiting times and patient satisfaction, for example. It had not been possible to undertake any literature review as nothing could be found in the literature to support the development of this unique system. Following detailed discussion and work within the team and discussion with stakeholders, the physiotherapy manager committed the system – including the capacity planning – to paper. The paperwork also underwent a series of further changes as the system was further developed and evolved; there is no 'finish point' in a dynamic development such as this.

- **Implementation**

Having completed the specification and all preceding stages the system was implemented in October 2003. This was the culmination of several months development work. However, the system continued through a further series of changes based on audit, feedback and evaluation over a long period. Authority to implement the system was based within therapy services and 'outside' permissions were not necessary.

- **Determine evaluation parameters**

Evaluation parameters were set and agreed to ensure that the change programme met the aims, objectives, direction and vision. The parameters agreed were: measurement of DNA rates, waiting list monitoring, assessment and measurement of number and content of complaints, formal audits of patients' views and level of satisfaction or otherwise, formal audit of those patients who did not contact the physiotherapy department (having been referred), formal audit of clinical outcomes, audits of referrer views and staff/team views.

All of these measures would be used to feed into further development to improve the system where necessary and to ensure that the change programme met the need of patients and all other interested parties.

Skills for success

- **Management skills**

The head of therapy services delegated responsibility for management and leadership of the change project to the out-patient physiotherapy manager who was accountable for the process. This included the delegation of authority to bring about the changes agreed within the team. The head of therapy services was fully committed to supporting the physiotherapy manager and his team through the process.

- *Strategic thinking skills* were essential to ensure that the overall vision and direction were maintained throughout.
- *Creativity* was required on the part of the whole team throughout the entire process; 'Choice Appointments' was a 'first' in the UK and a number of problem solving techniques and innovative ways of thinking were essential to the success of the project. Too often the pressures of daily patient care provision, managerial, financial and other important demands push managers into a reactive approach; however, the experience was that creativity and pro-activity can flourish if carefully lead.
- *Negotiating and influencing skills* were called upon throughout. For example, some team members were sceptical about the possible benefits of the new

system and resistant to the idea of 'surrendering' more control over episodes of physiotherapy care to patients. It was necessary to negotiate with these team members, ensure that their views were actively listened to and incorporated to influence views. There were also negotiations and influencing strategies to be used in discussion with GPs, commissioners and consultants for example.

- *New resources* were not required for this project; however, the physiotherapy manager was able to negotiate funding for a telephone system from voluntary sources and persuade the providing company to supply this at a favourable price.
- *Political skills* were needed for a basic understanding of the micro and macro contexts for introduction of the system and it was necessary to exercise political skills with a small 'p' and 'nouse'.
- *The management style* adopted ensured participation and team working, that all involved could participate fully in the development and that their contributions were valued and important. A variety of management styles were employed in different situations, where for example, decisions needed to be formalised and adhered to; responsibility having to be taken and authority to implement various phases at agreed times. The ability to adopt appropriate management skills and styles in different circumstances is an important attribute of management. The achievement of 'ownership' and participation is dependent on well managed and well led team working.

- **Leadership skills**
  - *Clear vision* and focus on the desired outcomes situation and commitment to ensuring that the service was patient-centred and provided a tangible improvement in quality of care were essential elements.
  - *Excellent communication* between all involved in the development and at all levels, all disciplines, groups and stakeholders involved was essential. Good communication is more that a 'two-way process', in order to achieve success all those with an interest should be included: as a consequence communication is multi-directional, not just two-way.
  - *Change often challenges our comfort zones* and this project was no exception as not all participants were equally enthusiastic or committed at the outset. Leadership and management skill needs to be exercised in challenging 'comfort zones' in a positive way in order to give time for the success of the project to reinforce advantages and benefits and 'win people over'. The challenging of 'comfort zones' often needs to take place, but in a positive manner.
  - *'Ownership'* of the project was ensured by full team participation in the development work which engaged all team members and thus empowered them in the re-design process.

Evaluation

- **Implementation within the agreed timescale** was achieved.

'Choice appointments' was unique, encompassing a totally new appointments system and new ways of working – giving more control to patients. As such, the system needs ongoing adjustments and further innovation in the light of experience, feedback from patients, staff and other stakeholders. Examples of changes implemented later have been the introduction of new paperwork to support the system, improved use of IM&T, refined capacity planning and so on.

- **The success criteria** were met and exceeded.
  - DNAs were reduced from 11.3% per annum to less than 1% within the first three months, saving capacity of 11.3% – time wasting is eliminated – with the result that staff are able to spend more time with patients, plan clinical related work effectively such as record keeping, team meetings and in-service training. Importantly capacity for taking more patients is increased.
  - Waiting times for non-urgent referrals were decreased from around 14–16 weeks to a few days only. During the first three and a half years there were no complaints about waiting times.

Early in 2006 another trust adopted the system with similar results, reducing DNAs from 17% per annum to less than 1%, waiting time from 12–14 weeks to a few days and liberating 22% greater capacity within the department. The bar charts at Figures 2.10, 2.11 and 2.12 illustrate these dramatic results for both services.

Formal audits have been undertaken in both services which indicate 94% patient satisfaction with the system (based on 100% questionnaire return, see Figures 2.13 and 2.14).

All these service improvement outcomes were achieved without any increase in resource input in financial terms although time and effort were invested in setting up the system.

Further audits including clinical outcomes have been put in place to ensure that views and feedback from patients, staff and stakeholders are incorporated into ongoing development.

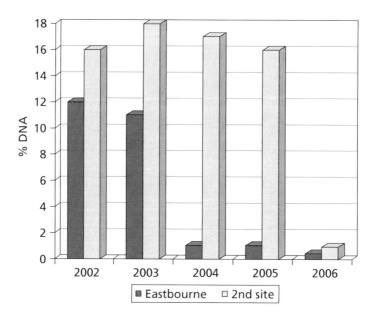

Figure 2.10 Percentage DNA.

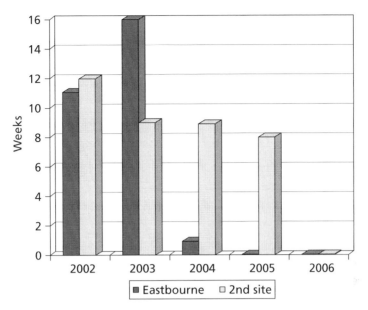

Figure 2.11 Routine waiting time.

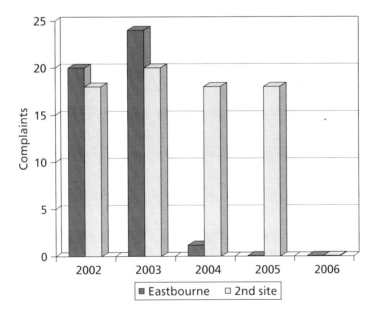

Figure 2.12 Waiting time complaints.

Learning points

In this case, as in all change management programmes, it is a dynamic environment in which the project is never fully completed as there is a continuing process of audit and feedback together with constant change taking place within the organisation and wider health economy. It is therefore important that the

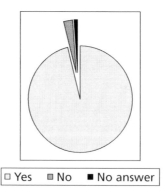

Figure 2.13 Was the information provided by the physiotherapy service appointment system clear?

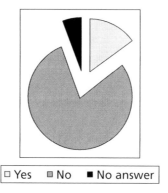

Figure 2.14 Would any other information have been useful?

system continues to develop in the light of the feedback, audit and other environmental changes taking place. However, following implementation of the system and having achieved the main aims and objectives, a process of reflection took place to assist learning from the experience and to incorporate lessons into other developments taking place and for the future.

- An understanding of the context in which the work took place in all its aspects was important to aid the development, vision, direction and implementation of the new system.
- Acknowledgement and understanding of constraints and barriers is essential so that strategies can be developed to overcome these, it is necessary to appreciate that it is not possible to improve or change all parameters surrounding the project.
- A clear vision of the desired situation – outcomes – helps cohesiveness of the team and ensures that everyone can be aware of, and sign up to, the overall aims and objectives.
- Involvement of people in the process from start to finish is crucial to success. All team members have important contributions which need to be listened to, understood and addressed, and incorporated. Thorough communication which

is timely, in all directions, clear, open and inclusive is essential. This will achieve 'ownership' and help to generate enthusiasm.

- Management support is essential at senior level to provide the multi-faceted back-up, ensure that the authority is delegated so that things can be made to happen, that managers and leaders involved in the project have responsibility for achieving the desired outcomes and are held accountable for the development appropriately. Senior managers also need to ensure that all the necessary infrastructures are in place to support the development.
- Resilience is needed on the part of all involved because things do not always go well or according to plan. Sometimes it is necessary to rethink the strategy, try another way or simply acknowledge and reject elements that do not give the positive answer envisaged.

Conclusions

- Sustainability: 'choice appointments' has been in place since the autumn of 2003 and has been highly acclaimed by patients. Audit of patients' views about the service gave very positive results on a 100% completion of the audit questionnaire by 355 consecutive patients over a six week period.

The system fulfilled all the original aims and objectives and is popular with referrers.

- Nationally: other services have adopted the system en bloc or elements of it. Feedback has been positive with significant interest in the system.
  - The National Health Service Institute for Innovation and Improvement (NHS III) has incorporated information about the system onto their website.[36]
  - More than fifty people have attended courses led by the out-patient physiotherapy manager on capacity planning and the implementation of 'choice appointments.'
  - The system was one of four national projects listed by the Public Sector People Management awards in 2006.
  - At the Institute for Health Improvement European Forum 2006 (Prague) the system was acclaimed by the IHI president as an 'outstanding example of a Kano Type 2 project. Excellent for patient care and introduced at no extra financial cost'.
- Locally: 'choice appointments' received the Trust award for innovations in excellent patient care 2005.

Case study 2 Stroke service re-design

In 2003 a service re-design of stroke services in South Devon was commenced using the framework for the management of change.

Moving from the current to the desired situation

- **Triggers for change**

Stroke was identified as the single greatest cause of long-term disability, with a marked increase associated with increasing age.

National targets and guidelines identified the need to ensure stroke services were providing best up-to-date care; the National Plan,[37] NSF for Older People,[38] Intercollegiate Working Party Guidelines.[39]

- **Managerial imperatives**

To redesign the service that would meet national targets, evidence-based care, user needs and commissioner requirements within an affordable financial framework.

- **Establish project group**

The project group was developed by the project lead to include representatives from: the healthcare multidisciplinary team from both acute and primary care organisations, patients, carers, social services operations managers, voluntary sector representatives, information department, public health analyst.

- **Shared vision, objectives and critical success factors**

The vision was developed to include several elements.
- Increase the number of patients who had suffered a stroke spending part of their stay on the stroke unit instead of being admitted to a general medical ward or never been admitted in the first place.
- Increase adherence to the hospital discharge policy.
- Increase number of patients accessing a CT scan within 48 hours.
- Increase number of stroke patients with record of being weighed while on stroke unit.
- Introduce direct booking for the Transient Ischaemic Attack (TIA) clinic.
- Improve primary care secondary prevention measures.
- Increase access to long-term support.
- Increase involvement of patients and carers in service improvement.

Essential actions

- **Data and information**

A wide range of data was collected and analysed. Problems were noted with coding. The information was used to inform the development of the project.

- **Timing**

A project plan was developed, supported by a GANTT chart, which was reviewed weekly.

- **Setting the direction**

A project launch was held, which was informed by the strategic plan developed by the project lead and CEO's of the organisations involved (one acute trust, two PCTs and two social service providers.)

- **Staff participation at all levels**

The project team included a wide range of staff of different organisations, different staff groups and different levels within the teams. For example a medical consultant was involved but also a ward clerk and a voluntary sector community based liaison officer.

- **Negotiation with stakeholders**

Stakeholders were kept informed at bi-monthly meetings about older people's services, when a briefing paper was included in the agenda, as well as one-to-one meetings as required – for example with finance directors.

- **Specification stage**

Once the current service had been reviewed along with the literature review and discussion with stakeholders it was possible to specify the model that was required to meet the needs identified in stage one.

- **Implementation**

This stage took nine months to reach. Following the specification it was necessary to gain strategic acceptance of the review recommendations which then gave authority to implement the proposed change to the stroke services.

- **Determine evaluation parameters**

In order to ensure that the change programme fitted the model of continuous improvement, evaluation parameters were set for monitoring and review and importantly to ensure that the change was sustained and further modifications made as necessary. The parameters included; length of stay in acute and community units, use of clinical outcome measures, access to TIA clinic, establishment of a thrombolysis service, ongoing input of user involvement.

Skills for success

- **Management skills**
  - The project lead was clear about the authority delegated to team members, identifying who had responsibility for which task and what action was required by a defined time.
  - Strategic thinking skills were required to ensure that the overall vision was maintained within the changing organisation situation that ensured over the nine months.
  - Creativity was required to solve problems and think laterally when difficulties were encountered. For example it was difficult to gather primary care information of secondary prevention measures so one GP practice was asked to develop a system that could gather the information required for the stroke review while ensuring that this complemented the work needed to inform GMS contract and QOF data.
  - It was necessary to use negotiating and influencing skills at many different levels, for example negotiating with organisations about a shift of care from secondary to primary care, developing more timely input for social services assessment and explaining the need to record patient weight to busy health care assistants.
  - Resources were needed at several levels. Time for staff to input to the project, skill mix and redeployment of staff following the review, funds to undertake minor works for the community unit to open, funding for the launch event.
  - Political awareness was needed to ensure that the project met key drivers in both health and social care.
  - The management style adopted ensured that as far as possible members felt included and valued, this aim helped to ensure that by being part of the project the members would own it and sustain the revised model.

- **Leadership skills**
  - There was a need for enthusiasm and commitment to ensure that the project succeeded. Working across health, social care and voluntary organisations required sustained commitment.

- A wide range of communication skills were deployed; formal briefing papers, team meetings, sub-group meetings, one-to-one meetings, formal presentations using graphs and data all ensuring that communication was meaningful with explanation and time for discussions and understanding.
- Comfort zones were sometimes challenged. This included bringing 'on board' those who were not keen to change the current service, as well as pressures caused by keeping to the project time scale.
- Sub-groups were established to ensure that staff of all levels were empowered and engaged in the service re-design.
- The concept of 'ownership' was captured initially at strategic level, ensuring the CEOs were committed, but also at team and individual level to ensure that all had input to the project which required them to report progress and implement small scale changes during the review. Service users and carers were essential, to inform the team of their experiences and views as well as a regular marker to measure whether the project was meeting their needs and desires.

Evaluation

The project concluded on time with a report to the strategic overview group. Criteria to measure sustainable success were agreed which included monitoring throughput, length of stay and quality measures. A training programme was put in place to support the development of the community service in particular, ensuring that acute unit and social care staff were included; reducing boundaries between different elements of the service.

Procedures were incorporated to ensure ongoing input from service users and expanding their roles as 'expert patients' to support other patients with stroke. The stroke review team meetings were replaced by stroke service meetings to include staff and users in regular evaluation and continuous service improvement which enabled subsequent developments such as the thrombolysis service and enhanced TIA clinic to be planned and monitored.

Learning points

Following the completion of the project the team reflected on the learning, with the aim of understanding what went well and where there had been difficulties. The purpose was to appreciate the hurdles which would inform methodology for future projects. The key points were:

- the context and timing was right. Having substantial evidence which confirmed there was room for improvement coinciding with an NSF priority which the organisations had committed to, was an ideal opportunity to implement a substantial change. If all organisations had not given commitment the change may not have occurred
- the constraints were imposed by factors outside the remit of the project. For example access to prompt CT scanning was a project running in parallel and requiring re-design of the imaging service, the access to this was an essential element of introducing thrombolysis. It was therefore agreed that this should be kept as a priority for future work. Financial constraints were expected and moving funds between organisations was not straight forward

- communication was the pivotal element requiring careful handling throughout the project. Poor communication leads to the 'grape vine'. Timing meetings well in advance so that staff could attend meetings was vital. Gathering data and sharing this with the project team was a powerful way of getting messages across
- co-ordinating the project required support from many services, information, finance, clinical departments and clerical support
- resilience. At times the project will not go according to plan, but keep enthusiastic and keep to the planned schedule.

Sustainable progress

There have been further changes following the implementation of the review. The information given to patients has been updated with user input which complements the stroke care pathway which was launched and updated two years later.

A community stroke unit was established under the leadership of an AHP consultant accepting patients who have been assessed and had immediate care at the acute hospital stroke unit.

Following the project the service has improved and been regularly audited. The percentage of patients, admitted to hospital with a diagnosis of stroke, able to be treated on the specialised stroke units has increased from 46% to over 82%. It has also:

- helped to ensure that any patients who are diagnosed with stroke but cannot be admitted to the stroke unit still receive specialised stroke care
- improved access to a specialised clinic for patients who have suffered suspected TIAs
- established a new thrombolysis service, so that suitable patients arriving at the hospital's A&E department can have rapid access to this service
- made it possible to organise therapy appointments ready for when the patient returns home from hospital, so that they know they have follow-up support already arranged
- prompted positive feedback from patients.

The stroke service has received a number of commendations:

- rated in the top five nationally by the Royal College of Physicians Sentinel Audit[40] for stroke care, and in the top two for service management
- cited as one of nine examples of good practice in stroke care by the Department of Health[41]
- featured in the NHS Primary Care Contracting PBC Bulletin on service redesign[42]
- selected as an example of good practice for provision of information to stroke patients by the National Stroke Association in its recent campaign 'Nobody Told Me'[43]
- winner of the 2006 Health and Social Care Award – improving access category.

Conclusion – change management

Change management describes a structured approach to transition. There are many roles and responsibilities for AHP managers in change management from recognising trends in the macro as well as in the micro-environment: change is a fact of life and not an option. The speed of change has increased dramatically in the NHS and society generally in recent years.

The world may not be spinning faster, but mankind certainly is.[4]

In this chapter we have shown that change management is not a distinct discipline with clearly defined and rigid boundaries, but that the theory and practice draws on a wide range of social science disciplines and traditions. The management of change has an extensive literature, being one of the most widely written about topics in the field of management. For this chapter we have selected a few of the many approaches, methodologies, techniques and models which we believe will be a useful guide for AHP managers.

We have also set out our own 'framework for the management of change' which is based on established change management theory and have presented case studies to demonstrate its practical application.

Change management cannot be seen in isolation as there is always interaction with the external environment as well as with internal sub-systems within organisations. It is important that change management incorporates careful and thoughtful planning and sensitive introduction and implementation including real consultation with, and involvement of, the people affected by the change as well as those involved in the re-design and implementation process. Sometimes managers will need to support staff to overcome negative thinking – which may present obstacles to change – embodied in phrases such as 'we've always done it that way'. Strong resistance to change may be rooted in deeply conditioned or historically reinforced feelings and practices and in this context it is important that managers are aware of the various stages typically involved when change is imposed:

Box 2.5 Reactions to change.

Denial – 'this can't be real' or 'this is not happening'
Anger – 'why our team?' or 'how can they do this to us?'
Bargaining – 'if I do this, you do that...'
Depression or defeat – 'this is going to happen'
Acceptance – move on

When change is forced on people problems generally arise. Change must always be realistic, achievable and measurable. Before embarking on change management projects it is essential to answer the questions:

1 what do we want to achieve with the proposed change?
2 do we need outside help in bringing about the change?
3 how and when will we know that the change has been successful?
4 how will staff, the service and organisation be affected by the change and how will they react?

It is important to remember that often the greatest insecurity for most staff is change itself, change may be disturbing and threatening. The manager has responsibility to facilitate and enable change and the behaviour of managers is crucial to the success of the process; for example some attitudes and behaviours can be counter productive such as the use of inappropriate language: 'We must change people's mindsets' or 'change people's attitudes'. Expressions such as these, are likely to signal imposed change. In order to achieve positive outcomes participation and involvement are essential with open, early and fully inclusive communication.

As we have indicated there are a number of clearly definable principles involved in successful change management including:

- always involve people and provide appropriate support
- understand where the organisation is at the moment – the current situation
- understand where you want to get to – the vision, desired situation
- understand when, why and what the measures and monitoring procedures will be
- plan development in appropriate, measurable stages
- communicate, involve, listen, enable and facilitate
- put relevant training programmes in place where necessary
- celebrate success
- evaluate, learn and readjust
- do not decide on the end before you begin.

There are many challenges and opportunities for AHP managers in the NHS to manage and lead change and to become involved in this important area of management practice; a positive, informed and systematic approach is essential for the achievement of successful outcomes.

Authors' note

The Authors acknowledge and would like to thank colleagues and staff in East Sussex and South Devon for their innovation and commitment to the illustrated change management programmes.

References

1 Heraclitus. In: *The Oxford Library of words and phrases. Vol 1 Quotations*. Oxford: Oxford University Press; 1981.
2 Johnson S. Of the laws of ecclesiastical polity. In: *The Oxford Library of words and phrases. Vol 1 Quotations*. Oxford: Oxford University Press; 1981.
3 Burnes B. *Managing Change – a strategic approach to organisational dynamics*. Harlow: Pearson Education Ltd; 2000.
4 Patton R, McCalman J. *Change Management – A Guide to Effective Implementation*. London: Sage Publications; 2000.
5 Iles V, Sutherland K. *Managing Change in the NHS. Organisational change a review for healthcare managers, professionals and researchers*. NCC SDO. 2001. www.sdo.lshtm.ac.uk.
6 Handy C. *The Empty Raincoat*. London: Hutchinson; 1994.
7 Handy C. *Understanding Organisations*. London: Penguin Business Books; 1999.
8 Hooper A, Potter J. *The Business of Leadership; adding lasting value to your organisation*. Aldershot: Ashgate Publishing; 2002.
9 Mintzberg H, Quinn JB. *The Strategy Process; concepts, contexts and cases*. New Jersey: Prentice-Hall; 1988.
10 Bennis W, Nannus B. *Leaders: strategies for taking charge*. New York: Harper Business; 1997.
11 Mullins L. *Management and Organisational Behaviour*. Harlow: Pearson Education Ltd; 2002.

12 Pond C. Leadership in the Allied Health Professions. In: Jones R, Jenkins F, editors. *Allied Health Professions – Essential Guides. Managing and Leading in the Allied Health Professions*. Oxford: Radcliffe Publishing Ltd; 2006.

13 Jones R, Jenkins F. *Allied Health Professions – Essential Guides. Managing and Leading in the Allied Health Professions*. Oxford: Radcliffe Publishing Ltd; 2006.

14 Hooper A, Potter J. *Intelligent Leadership*. London: Random House; 2001.

15 Burnes B. *Managing Change – a strategic approach to organisational dynamics*. Harlow: Pearson Education Ltd; 1996.

16 Obholzer A, Roberts V. *The Unconscious at Work: individual and organisational stress in the human services*. Hove: Brunner Routledge; 2000.

17 Baker A, Perkins D. Managing People and Teams. In: Glynn J, Perkins D, editors. *Managing Healthcare*. Canterbury: Saunders; 1995.

18 Pettigrew F, McKee, L. *Shaping Strategic Change*. London: Sage; 1992.

19 Schon D. *Beyond the Stable State*. New York: Lawton; 1971.

20 Lewin K. Groups Decisions and Social Change. In: Swanson G, Newcomb TM, Hartley EL, editors *Readings in Social Psychology*. New York: Holt, Rhinehart and Winston; 1958.

21 Schein E. *Organisational Culture and Leadership*. San Francisco: Jossey-Bass; 1992.

22 Handy C. *The Gods of Management*. London; Random House: 1991.

23 Schneider S, Barsoux J. *Managing across Cultures*. Harlow: Pearson Education; 2003.

24 Kotter J. *Leading Change*. Boston, Harvard Business School; 1996.

25 Wesley F, Mintzberg H. Visionary leadership and strategic management. In: Henry J, Walker D. *Managing Innovation*. London: Sage; 1999.

26 Potter J. *Introducing the Human Relations Aspect of Change*. Exeter University: Centre for Leadership Studies; 2002.

27 Goleman D. *Emotional Intelligence – why it can matter more than IQ*. London: Bloomsbury Publishing; 1996.

28 Goleman D. Leadership that gets results. *Harvard Bus Rev*. 2000; Mar-Apr: 79–90.

29 Katzenbach J, Smith D. *The Wisdom of Teams*. Boston: Harvard Business School Press; 1993.

30 Hirshhorn L. *The Workplace Within*. Cambridge: Massachusetts Institute of Technology; 2000.

31 Thakur M, Bristow J, Carby K. An Introduction to Organisational Development. In: *Personnel in Change*. Institute of Personnel Management; 1978.

32 Lippit R, Watson J, Priestly B. *The Dynamics of Planned Change*. New York: Harcourt Brace and Jovanovitch; 1958.

33 Saunders R. Communicating Change. In: *Managing Change to Reduce Resistance*. Boston: Harvard Business School Press; 2005.

34 Garvin D. *Learning in Action: A guide to putting the learning organization to work*. Boston: Harvard Business School Press; 2000.

35 Kotter P. Leading Change – Why transformation efforts fail. *Harvard Bus Rev*.1995; Mar–Apr: 59–67.

36 http://www.18weeks.nhs.uk/public/default.aspx?load=CaseStudies.

37 www.dh.gov.uk/.../OrganisationPolicy/Modernisation/NHSPlan.

38 www.info.doh.gov.uk/doh/oldpeople.nsf/.

39 www.rcplondon.ac.uk/college/ceeu/ceeu_stroke.

40 RCP Sentinel Audit. http://www.rcplondon.ac.uk/pubs/books/strokeaudit/.

41 http://www.dh.gov.uk/PolicyAndGuidance/HealthAndSocialCareTopics/OlderPeoples Services/OlderPeoplePromotionProject/OlderPeoplePromotionProjectArticle.

42 http://www.primarycarecontracting.nhs.uk/uploads/pbc_files/bulletin.

43 http://www.stroke.org.uk/campaigns/current_campaigns/nobody_told_me.

Chapter 3

Care pathways and the Allied Health Professional

Fiona Jenkins and Robert Jones

The link between AHPs and care pathways

AHPs provide healthcare in a wide variety of settings, for example hospital in-patient, out-patient, domiciliary, occupational health and schools. AHPs also work at different levels of authority ranging from undergraduate supervised practice through a range of autonomous clinical positions, expert and consultant practitioners and managerial posts. Whatever the profession, the place of work or grade of post, all AHPs have a duty to ensure that they provide the best possible service, which in turn requires them to deliver evidence-base care. Care pathways have been upheld by Roy[1] as:

> The key to unlocking the national agenda for improved services, increased responsibility, through clinical governance, and an easy route into the information superhighway.

The term 'integrated' tends to refer to a combined pathway of care and a multi-disciplinary documentation recording system. This chapter focuses primarily on the care pathway, although reference will be made to the all encompassing Integrated Care Pathway (ICP). The combination of high quality multi-disciplinary intervention underpinned by evidence-based practice is best provided through the use of the care pathway approach. For AHPs this can be translated to mean providing the best possible co-ordinated service for the patients by:

- streamlining the patient journey through health/social care
- doing the right things in the right order – the right patient at the right time and place, in the right way, with the right outcome
- clarifying role and responsibilities of the multi-disciplinary team
- involving patients in their own care
- ensuring that there is attention to the patient's experience
- developing appropriate patient information.

Clinical guidelines are often better at focusing on diagnosis and interventions than they are ensuring care is organised and effectively managed. Although patients are unique individuals they are often similar enough to warrant the development of guidelines based on evidence to improve both the co-ordination and the consistency of care. Historically the major focus of care pathways was the treatment of surgical patients in acute hospitals. However, there has been subsequent development of pathways that provide care in a range of settings and by a wider multi-disciplinary team. AHPs need to ensure that their interventions are co-ordinated with the rest of the health and social care teams – and that the patient is truly central to receiving the best care possible. One of the main challenges facing healthcare professionals and managers is the need to make the best use of limited resources, whilst providing high quality, timely, evidence-based practice.

Potential benefits from this approach often fail to be realised due to poor project planning and management.

> People and perfect processes make a quality health service – a poor quality service results from a badly designed and operated process, not from lazy or incompetent healthcare workers.[2]

Care pathways are a way of encouraging the translation of national guidelines into local protocols and their subsequent translation into local practice as well as a method for systematic gathering of clinical data for audit purposes.[3] As AHPs are involved in a wide spectrum of healthcare and provide interventions in diverse settings they are ideally placed to ensure that care pathways are used to provide the best care for patients and clients; they are equally well placed to help develop pathways themselves.

We have designed this chapter to provide a step-by-step guide to developing both the integrated and care pathway versions developed following practical experience of developing, implementing and monitoring multi-disciplinary pathways with reference to a theoretical base.

What is a care pathway?

A care pathway contains a number of different elements including planning, implementation, followed by ongoing review. The equivalent to pathways in industry would be called by other names, possibly a combination of good practice, quality control plus a large portion of ongoing quality improvement and design modification. In healthcare a care pathway is viewed as a multi-disciplinary outline of anticipated care. However, confusingly there is no single agreed definition of an ICP. A number of definitions have been in use since the late 1990s. Some confusion has been created because they all link ICPs directly to patient groupings or case-types. A single ICP rarely covers the full span of a patient 'journey' for a particular condition; the patient's care plan is commonly built up from a group of pathways, each of which describe a component or phase of the care for example an admission or assessment phase, a set of interventions and a discharge phase.

Definitions commonly quoted include:

1 the European Pathway Association:[4] care pathways are a methodology for the mutual decision making and organisation of care for a well-defined group of patients during a well-defined period. Defining characteristics of care pathways includes:
   - an explicit statement of the goals and key elements of care based on evidence, best practice, and patient expectations
   - the facilitation of the communication, co-ordination of roles, and sequencing the activities of the multi-disciplinary care team, patients and their relatives

- the documentation, monitoring, and evaluation of variances and outcomes; and the identification of the appropriate resources
- the aim of a care pathway is to enhance the quality of care by improving patient outcomes, promoting patient safety, increasing patient satisfaction, and optimising the use of resources.

2 Journal of Integrated Care:[5] an Integrated Care Pathway determines locally-agreed, multi-disciplinary practice based on guidelines and evidence, where available, for a specific client group. It forms all or part of the clinical record, documents care given and facilitates the evaluation of outcomes for continuous quality improvement.

3 evidence-based medicine:[6] a care pathway can be defined as a structured multi-disciplinary outline of anticipated care, placed in an appropriate time frame, to help a patient with a specific diagnosis or set of symptoms move through a continuum of care; receiving evidence-based care to maximise positive outcomes.

4 Wilson:[7] a multi-disciplinary process of patient focused care which specifies key events, test and assessments, occurring in a timely fashion to produce the best prescribed outcomes, within the resources and activities available, for an appropriate episode of care.

All the definitions emphasise that care pathways bring together evidence-based multi-disciplinary practice for a particular group of patients, to outline the optimum episode of care for all patients who have a specific condition or who are undergoing specific procedures.

The current most widely accepted definition in the UK has been developed by the National Pathways Association (NPA):[8]

Box 3.1 NPA definition of a care pathway.

An ICP determines locally agreed, multi-disciplinary practice based on guidelines and evidence where available, for a specific patient/client group. It forms all or part of the clinical record, documents the care given and facilitates the evaluation of outcomes for continuous quality improvement.

ICP's also known as co-ordinated care pathways, care maps or anticipated recovery plans, are essentially task orientated care plans which set out essential steps in the care of patients with a specific diagnosis or problem and describe the patient's intended clinical plan.[9,10] They are also useful in understanding why care sometimes falls short of locally adopted standards and can be a useful tool in supporting clinical audit and further service improvement.

The history and spread of care pathways

Critical path and process mapping methodology was used in industry, particularly in the field of engineering from as early as the 1950s. In the 1980s, clinicians in the USA began to develop the pathway tool within 'Managed Care'; re-defining the delivery of care and attempting to identify measurable outcomes. The focus was on the patient rather than the system, but needed to demonstrate efficient processes in order to fulfil the requirements of the insurance industry.

In the early 1990s the NHS funded a patient focused initiative to support organisational change, resulting in investigation and development of concepts such as pathways. In 1990 a team from the UK visited the USA to investigate the use of these pathways or 'Anticipated Recovery Pathways' as they were then called. As a result 12 pilot sites for pathways were set up in North West London in 1991–2. The West Midlands pathway development work commenced. By 1994 the Anticipated Recovery Pathway had evolved in the UK, care pathways were clinician led and driven and had patients and locally agreed best practice at the centre of their focus.

In response to demand for co-ordinated care pathway user groups, the National Pathways User Group – re-named the National Pathway Association – was set up in 1994; continuing until 2002. The NeLH pathways database and the International Web Portal,[11] were launched in 2002 to enable the free sharing of ICPs across the UK and to provide care pathway user and developer forums for discussion and sharing of best practice and development skills. Since 1992 care pathways have been developed and implemented across many healthcare settings in the UK – acute, community, primary, mental health, private, independent, NHS.

ICPs are now used all around the world including the USA, Canada, New Zealand, Australia, Germany, Belgium and the Netherlands.

Why develop care pathways?

There are many good reasons for developing pathways to provide a structured framework for both existing practice and developments. They:

- ensure the provision of consistent high quality care
- transfer evidence-based care into practice
- are patient centred, inclusive and clinically driven
- reduce unnecessary variation in practice
- reduce risk
- provide integration of care across organisational boundaries
- enable training/education and skills transfer
- are a tool for systematic action to facilitate continuous improvements in patient care
- provide evaluation of the impact of service re-design and improvement
- are a model to underpin many key local and national agendas simultaneously
- provide an opportunity to involve teams in service re-design.

The use of pathways can ensure the care process is better monitored and streamlined for the majority of people in a given patient or client population; providing patients with more consistent care and services, by minimising variations in practice. As they are based partly on previous clinical cases, providers are better equipped to predict all aspects of the care process including: milestones, complications, outcomes and improve the quality of care provided to the next patient with the same condition.

Care pathways help ensure a high degree of efficiently delivered care for a defined population. Once a pathway has been put in place, key indicators are regularly monitored to assess effectiveness. This information is used for learning rather than to judge individual performance and helps target areas in need of improvement.

What care pathways contain

- Algorithms defining the planned pathway within a time frame
- Referral, transfer and discharge guidance
- Local and national standards
- Evidence-based guidelines
- Patient information
- Information recording – this will make the care pathway a full ICP and will form all or part of the clinical record. For example, problem orientated medical record or similar structured freehand text area:
  - a system of review – variance tracking
  - tests, charts, assessments, diagrams, letters, forms, information leaflets, satisfaction questionnaires and so on
  - scales for measurement and outcomes of clinical effectiveness
  - 'space' to add activities or comments to a standard ICP to individualise care for a specific patient.

Care pathways and clinical governance

Care pathways provide defined standards and stages along the patient 'journey', they help reduce unnecessary variations in care, which may compromise clinical outcome. Pathways improve multi-disciplinary and multi-agency collaboration and importantly, empower patients and carers to be informed about and engaged in the care programme.

Many patients receive care that spans, not only health organisation boundaries, but also partner sectors such as education and social services. Working with organisations which mostly adhere to different governance principles may cause lack of clarity about lines of accountability. The Audit Commission[12] believes that it is vital that there should be clarity between partners regarding purpose, roles and responsibilities. The use of care pathways strengthens clinical governance procedures within organisations and across them.

The aim of care pathways

Patients whose care is organised and managed through pathways should be given realistic information about their healthcare as well as the likely progression of treatment and care. Involving patients will engage them actively, encouraging questions about prognosis and future healthcare needs, improving their satisfaction with services and reduce misunderstanding and complaints.

Box 3.2 The aims of care pathways.

- Provide best evidenced-based care
- Facilitate translation of national directives into local practice
- Improve multi-disciplinary and multi-agency communication
- Sustain and make equitable quality standards
- Reduce variance in practices
- Improve clinician/patient communication and satisfaction
- Identify research and development questions
- Involve team members in service development

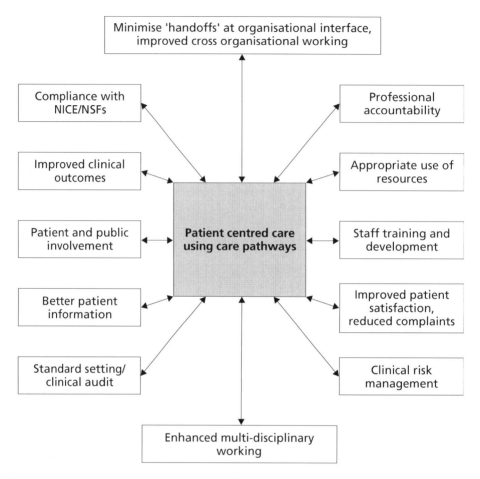

Figure 3.1 Integrated care pathways and clinical governance.

From the initial easily definable care pathways of the 1990s that addressed single procedures, there was an evolution of pathways that embraced the more complex conditions and ones that encompass not only in-patient healthcare, but also community and multi-agency care. With input from people with the appropriate range of skills, care pathways can be developed to ensure that optimum care is provided in every setting.

The ways in which care pathways have been developed vary; some people feel they should reflect the desired outcomes rather than only the current practice, because focusing on current ways of working may lack the impetus for change. Pathways should incorporate the evidence base with what is possible to provide locally with the resources available.

Some practitioners consider the documentation recording system alone to be the care pathway. This is a misconception which must be addressed at the outset of development. The pathway is often depicted as an algorithm, showing various routes that the patient may take on the 'journey' through their healthcare programme – and is the template on which future care delivery will be based. The way in which documentation is used to support the pathway is one of the elements of developing a full ICP. Many organisations choose to develop referral guidelines or pathways that include algorithms but exclude unified documentation systems. In practice both an algorithm of the care pathway and specifically developed documentation recording notes have been demonstrated to improve the quality of care, which requires best practice to be commissioned, provided and evaluated.

The healthcare team is likely to benefit from the use of care pathways. Clinical teams are able to develop their team working skills, which have been shown to improve patient care.[12] Additionally the relationship that exists between the professionals from different agencies involved in providing care for specific patient groups can be both defined and enhanced during the development of pathways. Each pathway should demonstrate commitment to:

- be patient centred
- cross professional and organisational boundaries
- be evidence-based
- form a single shared record of care – where a full ICP is developed
- be audited and modified in light of this
- include feedback from users.

Ten phases to developing care pathways

We propose ten phases for the development of a care pathway. There are several elements to be sequentially achieved in developing care pathways illustrated in Box 3.3. Each phase requires facilitation, management, decision making and team action.

Box 3.3 Ten steps to developing care pathways.

1   Choosing a clinical area.
2   Review the evidence.
3   Collect data and measure.
4   Review current practice including process mapping.
5   Identify key indicators.
6   Drafting the ICP.
7   Review and revise ICP draft.
8   Develop user version of care pathway.
9   Launching care pathways.
10 Monitor indicators, review and amend.

Phase 1: Choosing a clinical area

Selecting an important area of practice should be the first stage to address. A shared understanding of the organisation's strategic direction is essential, as is the commitment of senior management and clinical staff. A care pathway is, among other things, a change management tool and should be an integral part of the organisation's business and governance systems. The strategic 'vision' is imperative, which ensures that the whole team works towards a set of corporate aims.

Selection criteria could include common conditions; costly interventions, procedures where variations in practice occur and affect patient outcomes, those where there is a high level of interest, those with a changing evidence-base, or those areas which commissioners or providers of services identify suitable for attention and development.

The key tasks at this stage are:

- *define goals of the care pathway* – wherever possible, based on evidence of effective practice rather than, 'the way we do it round here'
- *team approach* – use a multi-disciplinary team approach. Steering group and working groups should comprise frontline staff, service users and additional people who have knowledge or expertise in the area
- *developing the team – steering committee* – recognise importance of reaching a common understanding of the function of the group and the parameters within which it will operate. Agree on timescales and communication processes
- *choosing a population, consider as high priority* – high volume, high cost, significant variability in practice, high morbidity/mortality, high public profile, reliance on multi-disciplinary team, demonstrated interest of carers to participate in the process
- *key stakeholders* – determine how to keep stakeholders informed and ensure their concerns are addressed
- *adapt or design?* – two main options are: adapt an existing pathway developed elsewhere or create your own. The National Electronic Health Library hosts a large database of existing ICPs, which should be consulted before designing your own.[11]

Whatever the 'prime mover' for identifying the need for a care pathway it is imperative that the identification of the topic is quickly followed by the appointment of the project team. Support for the project should be gained locally – from both commissioner and provider units – which must include the key healthcare team. To obtain engagement at an early stage is essential; the team needs a range of skills as outlined in Box 3.4.

Box 3.4 Project team members and skills.

- Management and leadership
- Clinicians involved in day-to-day delivery of care from a range of professional backgrounds
- 'Experts' familiar with current evidence-base
- Those providing diagnostic interventions
- Those providing rehabilitation services
- Service commissioners
- Financial modelling skills
- Patients/carers with experience of receiving care
- Project management skills
- Information management and data analysis skills
- Communication skills
- Audit skills for ongoing evaluation
- Support staff
- Facilitation skills

Phase 2: Review the evidence

The multi-disciplinary group needs to undertake a thorough review of the literature, identifying the evidence base on intervention and caring for the targeted population. The information should be assessed ensuring it meets the requirements for national guidelines and standards where these exist, for example NICE and NSFs as well as ensuring its relevance to local services.

It is important that some of the team members have skills in undertaking systematic literature reviews. A summary report highlighting key findings and recommendations from the reviewed literature must be drawn up and presented to the rest of the team.

Phase 3: Collect data and measure

The importance of accurate data cannot be over emphasised. Data is the keystone to understanding services and improving management of them. Time spent at an early stage collecting accurate, timely and relevant data will show rewards when analysis and audit of the service improvement is required later.

Measurement is fundamental to any model for service improvement. Having baseline information regarding current clinical practice is an important early step. The team needs to consider current practice rather than assumed practice. It is unlikely that any member of the project team will be fully informed of all the processes and procedures in place. It is important to maintain focus and collect only data directly related to the population under review. This may include economic data – length of stay, cost per case, income, number of episodes and contacts – as well as qualitative data from patients and carers.

Gathering data often requires extending the review team to include people experienced in coding and analysis. The complexity is compounded when data gathering extends across organisations and more so if it is needed from other agencies. Sources may also include case note reviews, public health and census statistics and organisational strategic development plans. Time spent on this exercise is well invested and not a stage that can be missed or compromised.

Measurement – what to measure?

Measurement is an essential part of the process. It is important to develop aims before measuring and to design measures around the aims. Also have clear definitions of measures and measure points, by:

- establishing a reliable baseline
- tracking progress over time
- collecting accurate and complete data
- making results available and feeding back.

Measurement should be used to expedite improvement. It is therefore important to select measures that:

- focus directly on the service being re-designed
- are designed around local and national aims and requirements
- are specific and clearly defined – specific, measurable, achievable, realistic, timed – SMART

- are pragmatic – add value, practical to collect and can be integrated into the daily routine
- are locally agreed and 'owned', not imposed
- incorporate experience from other services where appropriate
- obtain 'buy in' from local stakeholders
- link to improvement work with other initiatives in the health community
- meet requirements of clinical audit and clinical governance.

It is necessary to strike a balance between measures that are feasible to collect and measure the impact of the process change being tested and introduced.

Collecting data

The first stage is to define the starting point or baseline. This will require sufficient time before the improvement work begins. By doing this it is possible to demonstrate where changes have been beneficial. If no historical data exists it is important to commence measurement as soon as possible to establish a baseline.

It is a requirement to agree targets that the team wants to achieve and set up a system to monitor progress regularly. The targets must be linked to the aims and objectives agreed. Poor quality data can invalidate the development process. In order to improve data quality it is advisable to use it early on in the project – only then will it start to improve.

Use existing data wherever possible. It is important to ensure accuracy, timeliness, relevance, completeness and consistency for it to be used effectively. It may be necessary to collect the information manually at first. This is the case in many improvement initiatives and gives the chance to learn about the data collection process to ensure that it can be maintained in the longer term.

Sampling is the process of selecting a small representative group in order to draw conclusions about the population or cohort as a whole; this can be a useful technique. A sampling method that minimises bias should be chosen.

When selecting sampling methodology consider the following factors:

- clinical conditions
- process groups
- age groups
- gender
- time of day/day of week
- sampling technique for example, random, stratified or a given number.

Once measures have been agreed and data collected it will be necessary to analyse and present the data to others in the organisation.

A key to successful presentation of information is 'keep it simple'. Charts or diagrams need to be easy to understand. Ideally each element of the presentation should convey one message. Further information on measurement in healthcare is widely available.[11,13,14]

Understanding data collection, analysis and use for AHPs is discussed in detail in the next book of this series *Managing Money, Measurement and Marketing*.

Phase 4: Review current practice including process mapping

There are several methods of implementing change which we have presented and discussed in Chapter 2. The method most widely used in the development of care pathways is process mapping and the model for improvement. This was specifically adapted for use in healthcare by the Institute for Healthcare Improvement in the USA,[15] led by Langley et al.[16] The model was subsequently introduced into the NHS by the Modernisation Agency,[17] as one of their tools for service improvement.

The model for improvement was designed to provide a framework for developing, testing and implementing changes leading to sustainable improvement. It promotes the concept of small-scale study to make bigger sustainable changes. Its framework includes three key questions with a process for testing change ideas using 'Plan, Do, Study, Act' (PDSA) cycles. There are four stages to a PDSA cycle shown in Figure 3.2.

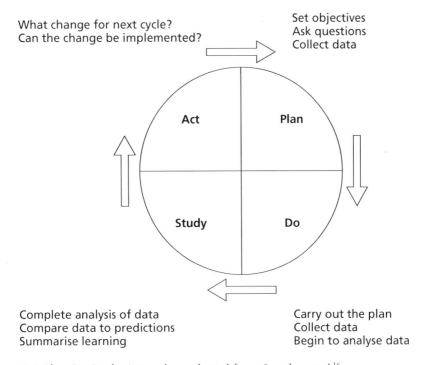

What change for next cycle?
Can the change be implemented?

Set objectives
Ask questions
Collect data

Act

Plan

Study

Do

Complete analysis of data
Compare data to predictions
Summarise learning

Carry out the plan
Collect data
Begin to analyse data

Figure 3.2 Plan Do Study Act cycle – adapted from Langley et al.[16]

The model has been shown to offer the following benefits:

- it is a simple approach
- it reduces risk by starting small – of particular importance when bringing about changes to clinical systems or care processes
- it can be used to help plan, develop and implement change
- it supports rapid cycles of improvement
- it can be highly effective

- it supports a 'bottom up' approach to change consistent with systems of continuous improvement
- it can also be used to facilitate large scale strategic plans.

There are many other successful models of service improvement which may be better suited for ICP development. These are further explored in Chapter 2.

Phase 5: Identify key indicators

Key indicators are milestones against which to measure progress along a care pathway. They are based on current literature and show where clients should be at specific stages in their care. Indicators must be monitored on a regular basis to ensure an individual is receiving optimum care. The Canadian Council on Health Services Accreditation[18] defines indicators as:

> Measurements, screens, or flags used as a guide to monitor, evaluate, and improve the quality of care, clinical services, support services, and organisational functions that affect client/client outcomes.

Indicators alert the service provider when the activity has reached an acceptable/unacceptable level; for example, waiting times. Indicators may be used as points of reference for evaluation and comparison. They can also be used to examine trends over time. Measuring and reporting of indicators encourages better services, which in turn will improve health outcomes. They are not used for evaluating the performance of individual staff members.

There are three types of indicators: Structure, Process and Outcome shown in Box 3.5.

Box 3.5 Types of key indicators.

- **Structure indicators** reflect the environment where the service is provided.
These indicators measure the characteristics of care or resources used to provide services to patients. They include the physical facilities, administrative organisation and qualifications and experience of staff. Environments with good structural properties normally provide quality care and service

- **Process indicators** reflect the way in which the service is provided.
These indicators measure the delivery of care or activities used to provide the service. They include the degree to which the services conform to the standards and expectations of the patient and the provider.

- **Outcome indicators** reflect the achievements of the delivered service.
These indicators or measures record the result or end products of care such as levels of mobility and functional ability. They measure the extent to which a desired change, effect or result was achieved for a patient.

It is important to select the appropriate indicators before the pathway implementation. Monitoring systems need to be set up to collect the range of indicators so that progress can be monitored as a routine rather than as an additional activity.

Phase 6: Drafting the care pathway

Algorithm

At this stage the process of care is analysed and modified to ensure that it is evidence-based and supported by the multi-disciplinary team providing care, other service providers, patients/service users and carers. During this analysis, it is likely that a decision making process will require clarification at some point in the care process. To ensure that the whole team clearly understands the defined process, an algorithm – decision making tree – should be produced. Algorithms are designed to guide practitioners through the 'if X, then Y' decision making process, which will guide them through the agreed route for intervention to be provided. This in turn ensures that patients are provided with consistent care. Though the algorithm defines the expected pathway for the majority of patients, there is scope for clinical judgment to determine an appropriate deviation from the pathway. An algorithm for Parkinson's disease is shown in Figure 3.3, and for back pain in Figure 3.4

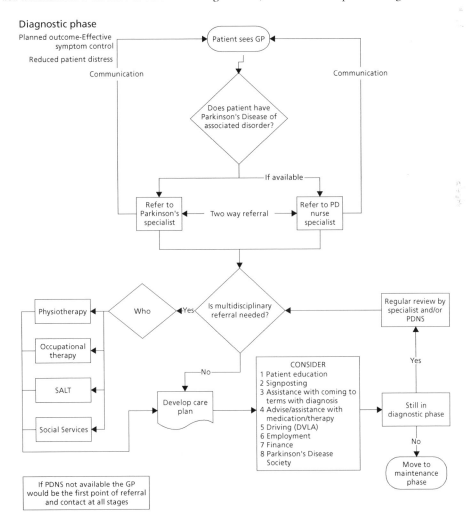

Figure 3.3 An example of an ICP algorithm for Parkinson's disease.

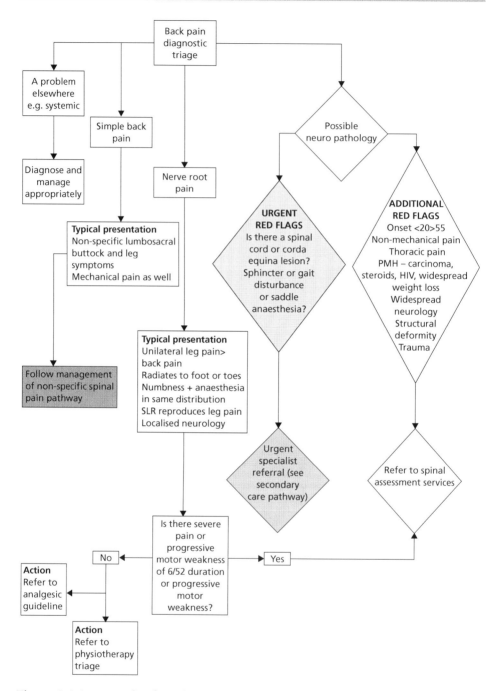

Figure 3.4 An example of an algorithm for back pain.

ICP documentation

Once the care pathway algorithm is agreed, it is possible to proceed to construct a single record of documentation. This includes the multi-disciplinary plan and care record which incorporates evidence-based recommendations and indicators

– developing a full ICP. All staff involved in the care process will need to contribute to integrating all relevant information from existing documentation. The scale of this task should not be underestimated. The difficulty of developing paperwork that meets the needs of all professional groups and organisations involved can be enormous. Electronic patient records that cross health, education and social care will, in time, radically change the way that information is recorded, stored and shared. However, it is necessary to develop paper-based systems in the interim.

Thorough documentation at the outset will avoid the danger of double recording, ensure accurate record keeping and that pathways meet the organisation's records requirements. The primary documentation form can be used by all members of the care team. It is necessary to ensure that the components of the pathway track the continuum of care – from initial assessment, to care provision and rehabilitation – in both secondary and primary care settings. To enhance and improve the efficiency of the ICP it is advisable to develop supporting paperwork such as standard procedures, and patient information and education materials, as shown in Box 3.6. The documentation may be either 'patient-held' or of the more traditional 'organisation-held' type. The 'patient-held' record should be used by staff and patients to record key information. This might include appointment details, individual goals, medication use diary, strategies and contingency plans. This record is used to inform the ongoing monitoring and evaluation of the individual's care.

Box 3.6 Items for consideration when developing ICP documentation.[19]

A single record of client care
Standard format
Simple in design and easy to follow
Consent
Abbreviations explained if used
Include realistic goals, timeframes and measurable outcomes
Provide an audit tool
Wording and content
Written in plain language
Include client information
Highlight roles and accountabilities
Include signatures of staff
Dynamics and flexibility
Incorporate guidelines, protocols and standards
Follow a logical sequence ensuring no duplication
Easy to complete
Easy to find relevant information
Variations recorded together with related actions

Phase 7: Review and revise ICP draft

Once the pathway has been developed it must be tested before proceeding to full implementation. The final testing enables feedback and suggestions for revisions from other representatives of all relevant disciplines. This input, however, must be considered carefully. If the comments received at this stage deviate from the evidence regarding best practice, it may be necessary to update and inform providers about recommended practices and the research evidence. Testing the revised version of the pathway with a small sample will help identify any further process, design, or system changes required before wider implementation. During this stage collection of a sample of key indicator data should also be undertaken to check that the care pathway works as intended.

Phase 8: Develop user version of care pathway

A user version of the pathway is a useful way to educate and involve patients in the care process. It also provides an opportunity to answer some of the common

The Stroke Care Pathway is designed to be used by the doctors, nurses and therapists who will be taking care of you, the patient, wherever you receive your care (at home, or in either acute or community hospital). This Patient's Version of the Care Pathway is identical, except without a lot of the medical jargon. You should be able to follow what is planned for your care by following the arrows as they lead from one box to the next (see Figure 3.5). The Pathway gives guidance for both clinicians and patients at the main decision points, but it is not intended to provide 'rules' for everything that might happen – that would be impossible, and there may be very good reasons why any particular treatment in your individual case is different. If you are concerned about what is happening or what might happen next you should always try to discuss this with your doctor, nurse or therapist – they will want to know what is worrying you.

As the process of stroke care develops this care pathway will be updated. For comments and feedback contact the xxxx

Some common questions people ask about stroke and Transient Ischaemic Attack (TIA)

What is a stroke?

A stroke is an illness in which part of the brain is suddenly severely damaged or destroyed. This causes a loss of function of the affected part of the brain. It usually causes weakness, paralysis of the arm and leg on either the left or right side of the body, twisting of the face, and in some cases other effects which may include loss of balance, disturbance of vision, disturbance of speech, loss of control of the bladder and bowels, and difficulty in swallowing. In very severe cases, there is a loss of consciousness or confusion of thought. The damage in the brain is caused by a blood clot or a haemorrhage.

What is a transient ischaemic attack ('TIA')?

A transient ischaemic attack or TIA is very like a stroke except that it passes quickly; the symptoms of weakness of one side of the body, tingling and twisting of the mouth or loss of speech or disturbance of vision last only for a few minutes or hours and then disappear. TIAs occur because, for a short time, not enough blood reaches part of the brain. They can be treated and anyone who experiences a TIA should see their doctor.

What is the risk of another stroke?

Life is a risky business, and if we thought about risk the whole time we would never cross the road or go up in an aeroplane. While there is no good reason to assume that one stroke will inevitably be followed by another, the condition that caused the first – such as high blood pressure – will need treating to reduce the chances of the same condition causing another stroke. After an ischaemic stroke (see box, top right), you will be prescribed aspirin to reduce the risk of another stroke.

It is best to try to train oneself to treat the fear of another stroke in the same way as you treat the danger of a crash when you buy an air ticket - it could happen, yes, but it probably won't.

Why should I have a six-month check-up?

It is strongly recommended that six months after your stroke, wherever you are living by then, you go back to your doctor or nurse at the surgery or health centre for a check-up. The doctor or nurse will want to check on your recovery from the stroke; they will want to check your medication and to see that everything is being done to reduce your risk of another stroke; and to see whether there is any need for more therapy for you.

What causes a stroke?

Most strokes occur in the second half of life and are caused by damage to the blood vessels – and sometimes to the heart – which has been building up slowly for many years. Most strokes happen when a blood clot forms in a damaged vessel and blocks the flow of blood to part of the brain (an *ischaemic* stroke), but some happen when a damaged blood vessel in the brain bursts and blood pours from it into the brain itself (a *haemorrhagic* stroke).

In at least half of all strokes the reason why the blood vessels become damaged in the first place is because they have been exposed to high blood pressure. If in addition the patient smokes, drinks heavily, is over-weight, takes too much salt in their diet, or has heart disease or diabetes the risk of stroke is increased. A number of other factors are suspected, but there is no single cause of stroke, and some strokes even happen without a cause ever being found.

Anyone can suffer a stroke at any time, although the risks can be substantially reduced by a healthy life style, including the avoidance of smoking, and especially by having your blood pressure checked and, if it is too high, ensuring that it is kept under control by treatment.

Why should I go to a Stroke Unit instead of my local hospital?

Research work over the last thirty years shows that people with stroke stand a better chance of surviving if they are cared for on a Stroke Unit. They also stand a better chance of recovering well enough to return home after the stroke. Because of this, the NHS runs a specialist Stroke Unit at the local hospital for the 'acute' period of care (generally the first week), so almost all people with stroke would go there first. After that, care is provided in the Stroke Rehabilitation Unit, or in your local community hospital. There, treatment and rehabilitation will continue, and if all goes well, plans can be made for your return home. If you need it, therapy can continue after you get home with therapists who can see you either as an out patient or in the community.

How can I get more information?

You should find that most of your questions about stroke and TIA can be answered by the health staff who are looking after you. Information can also be obtained from the Stroke Association, an independent national charity for people after a stroke and their carers, which runs telephone helplines and provides publications and welfare grants, and has affiliated local stroke clubs. The national website is www.stroke.org.uk. This Patient Version of the Care Pathway has been prepared with the help of local stroke patients and the Stroke Association.

Figure 3.5 An example of patient produced information.

questions patients are likely to have about their plan of care and various interventions. Using clear language to explain the various steps in the pathway, their projected timing and where appropriate provide key contact names and telephone numbers for further information. User versions are best developed by users themselves. Examples are shown in Figures 3.5 and 3.6.

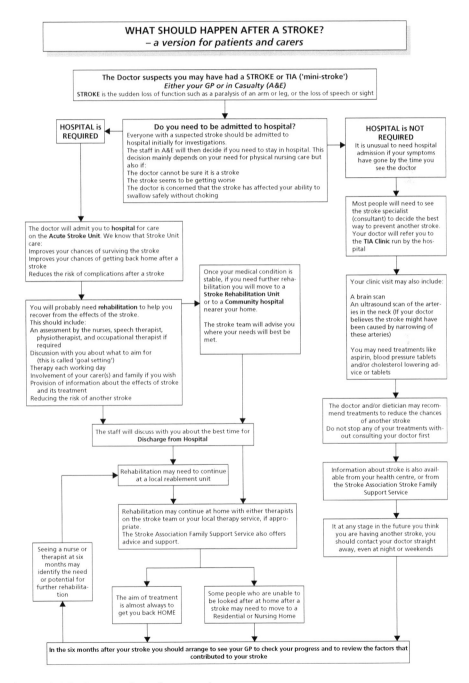

Figure 3.6 Patient version of care pathway.

Phase 9: Launching care pathways

The launch of an ICP will have a significant bearing on its success. A poorly launched care pathway will not be well used or adhered to and therefore have limited impact on patient care. It is essential to plan the launch as part of the project planning, this is one of the most essential milestones and where it is necessary to engage a much wider audience than during the developmental stages. The pathway will have a much greater impact if time is spent ensuring that those people who will use it in their day-to-day work understand the benefits and do not see it as 'just another pathway'. A robust launch strategy will improve the chances of successful implementation.

The strategy should identify the key stages of implementation and actions. The strategy should offer a checklist of tasks that are shared out among the implementation group.

- **Communication**: it is vital that people who will be asked to work in a different way following the introduction of the pathway are supported. Many good pathways falter due to the concerns of staff, who may regard the pathway as an imposition threatening their clinical freedom. The pathway may require staff to work with some agencies or services for the first time. It is important to the implementation to invest time in discussing and understanding the issues around professional regulation and accountability as well as exploring areas of commonality. Provide time in the implementation strategy to explore fully the potential benefits of the care pathway with the people who will be asked to implement it and the service users who will experience it. A key 'selling' point is the underlying objective to improve the quality of care which is evidence-based.
- **Awareness**: all staff using the pathway require information about the practical aspects of implementation. In addition the executive teams need to be made aware of the care pathway and its launch in order to ensure support at Board level. All relevant staff should have access to awareness sessions or briefings covering the principles of the pathway; the practicalities of how to work within it and how to make the most of it.

  It is often difficult to get everyone together at the same time to provide a formal awareness session. Multiple methods for briefing should be considered. These may include for example:
  - a formal launch at an event solely planned to begin the use of the new pathway. This is a good way to get a large group of staff together but it will be impossible to gather everyone who need to be aware of the ICP
  - 'road shows' where a few members of the steering group go to meet key staff at, for example, departmental meetings, practice meetings or voluntary organisations meetings
  - putting the care pathway onto a web page
  - e-mailing the pathway to key contacts
  - writing the pathway onto a CD
  - making paper copies available and sending to named individuals.
- **Timing:** ensure the launch of the ICP doesn't clash with other events which may detract from the impact of the launch.
- **Resources**: ICP development requires significant resource input especially in staff time. The launch itself will also need to be funded, do not under estimate

the administration time required. It is important to invite a wide range of people, for example, pathway users, carers, commissioners, the multi-disciplinary team, voluntary sector, communications leads. Record the names of all those who attend the launch sessions as gaps in representation can subsequently be followed up. There may be costs for room hire, refreshments, printing, copying and so on. Sponsorship can be mutually advantageous, but will depend on local circumstances and procedures.

Documentation

An integral part of all care pathways is thorough documentation. However, some pathways do not incorporate specifically designed multi-disciplinary record keeping system, but many do. The principles of good quality documentation and record keeping apply equally to ICPs as they do to traditional recording systems. Middleton and Roberts[19] report that there is consensus regarding ICP documentation, which should be:

- sequential, specifying timing and indicators how to move along the pathway
- written in plain language, avoiding abbreviations where possible.

They further suggest that there are two reasons why new documentation is likely to take more time to complete, neither of which is likely to continue in the long term.

1 Any new system requires familiarisation time. The act of having to turn pages over to find where to write a particular piece of information rather than writing it down on the next piece of blank paper will be more time consuming until staff are able to turn to the required place automatically.
2 ICPs may require some staff to write more than they did before, particularly in situations where previous documentation was not well completed and where routine notes about patients' progress were not kept to an adequate standard.

ICP documentation must meet the requirements of the legal care record, which can be challenging particularly when some care may be provided away from where the notes are held. For this reason some services implement ICPs without integrating record keeping systems. However, it is recommended that wherever possible a single record of care should be implemented. The electronic patient record will in time facilitate the use of one clinical record for all staff.

Decreasing the administrative burden for health and social care staff is a welcome by-product of a well structured ICP. Documentation is concerned with anticipating the 'routine' of care thereby guiding the practitioner to follow what is anticipated. Although the content of individual ICPs differs there are benefits to be gained by keeping to a standardised format. This might include:

- front page for patient details such as name and demographic information
- consent
- clinical assessment – including risk assessment
- care plan and patient management notes – which may be colour coded for ease of navigation.
- discharge planning
- variations from the expected pathway.

Comprehensive advice on the design of care pathway documentation is provided by de Luc.[20]

Phase 10: Monitor indicators – review and amend

It is important to establish a system for monitoring indicators in the care pathway. The method used depends on the stage of the pathway development and processes or outcomes being monitored.

- Implementation evaluation: in the initial stages of implementation it may be necessary to frequently monitor several of the intended pathway indicators to identify problems in the pathway itself. Once the pathway is established and implementation issues have been resolved, it can then be evaluated and revised to reflect new evidence and 'best' practices.
- Individual patient progress: these indicators relate to individual patients' progress along the pathway. Variations in the expected course at any stage will have implications for subsequent steps in the care process.
- Patient group outcome: these indicators relate to the entire group for which the pathway has been developed. These outcomes help identify 'bottlenecks' and constraints facilitating quality of care reporting, for example waiting times and length of stay.

Evaluation of care pathways

Analysis and review are essential processes in the evaluation of the effectiveness of care pathways. This also contributes to the cycle of continuous improvement and ensures that care and interventions are based on current evidence of effective practice.

Not only do indicators need monitoring, but the pathway itself needs maintaining. Pathways will continually evolve. If the care pathway is going to be used to promote continuous service improvement resources including staff need to be assigned to this work.

To maintain momentum, de Luc[20] suggests elements which need to be put in place.

Table 3.1 Checklist for pathway maintenance.

1 Nominate a person to lead the maintenance process
2 Ensure arrangements in place for production of revised pathway and updating
3 Where a paper recording system is used ensure on-going supplies
4 Nominate a care pathway trainer
5 Put in place training programme for new staff and updates for existing staff
6 Ensure staff are monitored for accuracy and timeliness of completing pathway
7 Set up an audit plan
8 Set dates for audit meetings for the multi-disciplinary team
9 Agree review date for the care pathway content, including user views

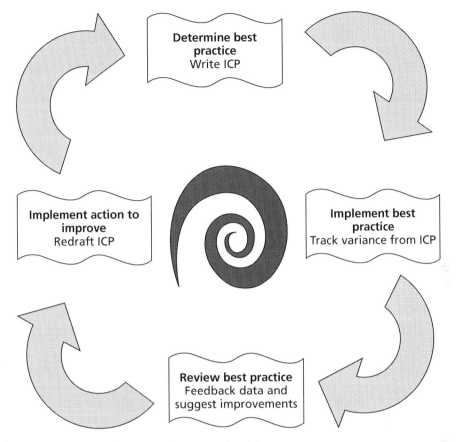

Figure 3.7 A care pathway continuous cycle of improvement.

The purpose of analysis and review

Before commencing the process it is necessary to identify several key indicators including:

- has the implementation of this pathway improved patient care?
- has it provided at least the same level of care at no more cost than previously?
- are there any changes that can be made which will improve its effectiveness?

It is also important to identify learning points arising during the course of a pathway, particularly those issues around partnership and collaborative working.

Middleton and Roberts[19] identify a number of possible areas to examine during a care pathway review:

- changes in documentation, that is accuracy, completeness, amount of time required to complete
- changes in care provision or process of care, for example introduction of guidelines, increased consistency, length of stay, number of contacts, shortening time delays, reducing number of contacts, changes in who provides care
- changes in patient and staff satisfaction
- changes in outcomes of care.

How to use care pathways

Once a care pathway has been developed all staff are expected to implement it. This will require them to:

- follow the care pathway for every patient within the specified care group
- use appropriate documentation and record interventions and pathway progress
- justify any deviation from the pathway and indicate the reasons for variation
- take appropriate action when progress deviates from that anticipated in the pathway
- ensure patients and carers understand the pathway and its application to them.

Benefits and barriers

Some of the possible benefits and barriers to successful implementation of care pathways are listed in Box 3.7. If the benefits do not outweigh the barriers then it

---

Box 3.7 Benefits and barriers to care pathway implementation.

Key benefits
1 Facilitate the introduction of protocols based on evidence
2 Promote more patient centred care – improving patient involvement
3 Facilitate inter-disciplinary working
4 Improve care planning and monitoring
5 Improve multi-disciplinary audit
6 Enable changing evidence-base to be quickly incorporated into practice
7 Identified areas for individual clinician improvement
8 Identified areas for whole service improvement
9 Make better use of resources
10 Improved service attracts more business
11 Improved record keeping
12 Improved Clinical Governance
13 Provides equity of access and care
14 Consistency and simplicity of commissioning
15 Quality assured services

Possible barriers
1 Appear prescriptive
2 Reduce clinical freedom
3 Be a resistance to change
4 Appear to be a cost saving initiative rather than one of quality improvement
5 Be difficult to obtain staff engagement and 'ownership'
6 Unrealistic time frame
7 Obstructive interpersonal politics
8 Fail to be adopted if communication is poor
9 Require significant service re-design
10 Require investment of resources
11 Lack leadership and project management skills
12 Not gain commissioner support
13 Conflicting organisational priorities

may indicate that the wrong clinical area is being addressed. There has been a lot of evaluation of ICPs with more than 4000 international references to the use of them and more than 45 different care group or diagnosis related pathways in use in the UK.[3] In addition to the benefits listed, there are reported additional benefits of improved patient outcomes, quality of life and reduced complications,[21] reduced length of stay in hospital, increased patient satisfaction,[19] reduction of cost of care,[22] improved inter-disciplinary communication and reduction of time taken by staff to complete paperwork. The latter point is worthy of note; as many clinicians consider at the outset, that note keeping time will be increased. However, due to the multi-disciplinary nature of the care pathway, duplication of assessment is significantly reduced, resulting in overall less time required for record keeping.

The barriers are not insurmountable. However, it is essential to recognise the importance of some of these; because if they are not addressed they may impede progress or prevent completion of the pathway. Clinician resistance can be a major barrier to pathway development and implementation. Recognising that the change process gives rise to question the way that care is currently provided – suggesting that current practice is not optimal – is an important factor. Skilful leadership is necessary to gain support from those staff keen to make the required changes, without alienating those who are slower to adapt and engage. Initially it is better to work with a small group of enthusiasts, rather than trying to persuade the wider team that the change programme is of value. One-to-one work with 'resistant' clinicians will give opportunity to find common ground and is a tactic worth exploring.

If, for example, significant service re-design is required to implement the new pathway and the timing is not right to embark on a major project, it might be better to delay implementation rather than fail. Therefore awareness of the possible barriers aids selection of the right care pathway to develop. Undoubtedly it is better to do this at the beginning of the process rather than at the end.

Conclusion

There is strong evidence that the experience of health professionals both in the UK and USA points to benefits of using care pathways.[23] For pathways to be successfully adopted they must be accurately completed and audited. Any deficiencies uncovered need to be remedied during the review stage. This rigor ensures that pathways remain 'live' processes fulfilling the purpose of providing evidence-based care for patients.

Arguably the best examples of care pathways tend to have several things in common, they frequently:

- examine the best evidence; locally, nationally and internationally
- use local knowledge, experience and expertise
- involve service users in the design and evaluation processes
- involve a number of different disciplines in a team decision; creating 'ownership'
- use continuous improvement models
- ensure teams have information for feedback on a regular basis
- review and amend the pathway in light of audit results or changing evidence-base and feedback.

There is a wealth of information available to assist, inform and guide pathway developers.[1, 8, 10,14,15,17,18,24,25,26,27,28,29]

There are however criticisms of ICPs and it is recognised that there is a need to develop more evidence about their effectiveness. McDonald and Paul[22] assert that:

> ICPs are helpful in achieving consensus on the consistency and continuity of care and can improve the documentation of evidence-based and patient focused care. ... the standard of ICPs is variable and, although their use is now widespread, they have not been meaningfully evaluated. Failures to identify improvements in care, following the introduction of an ICP have been linked to their implementation and variability in content quality. Although there are a large number of integrated care pathways listed on the National Electronic Library for Health, no 'kite mark' has been used to assure a sound clinical, managerial, ethical and legal footing for them.

Care pathways are reported to result in the provision of better quality care and almost always manage to do this at lower cost.[1] Cost containment itself may be a benefit, but equitable better quality care should remain the key objective. AHPs are an essential staff group in the development of care pathways and we advise AHPs to embrace the concept of care pathways, contributing their management, leadership and clinical expertise by participating fully in the design and implementation process.

References

1 Roy S. Foreword. In: De Luc K, editor. *Developing Care Pathways – the handbook.* Oxford: Radcliffe Medical Press; 2001.
2 http://www.jr2.ox.ac.uk/bandolier/Extraforbando/Forum2.pdf . 2003.
3 Campbell H, Hotchkiss R, Porteous M. Integrated care pathways. www.the-npa.org.uk.
4 European Pathway Association. Slovenia Board Meeting. December: 2005. http://www.e-p-a.org/index2.html.
5 Overill S. A practical guide to care pathways. *Int J Integr Care.* 1998; **2**: 93–8.
6 www. evidence-based medicine.co.uk.
7 Wilson J. *An introduction to multi-disciplinary pathways of care.* Newcastle: Northern Regional Health Authority; 1992.
8 www.the-npa.org.uk.
9 Coffey R, Richards J, Remmert C, *et al.* An introduction to critical paths. *Qual Manag Health Care.* 1992; **1**: 45–54.
10 Kitchiner D, Davidson C, Bundred P. Integrated care pathways; effective tools for continuous evaluation of clinical practice. *J Eval Clin Prac.* 1996; **2** (1): 65–9.
11 www.nelh.shef.ac.uk/nelh/kit/cps/paths.nsf/FO1?open.
12 Audit Commission. *Governing Partnerships. Bridging the Accountability Gap.* London: HMSO; 2005.
13 Campbell H. Integrated care pathways increase use of guideline. bmj.bmjjournals.com/cgi/content/full/317/7151/147/b.
14 http://www.venturetc.com/eicps.asp.
15 The Institute for Healthcare Improvement, USA. www.ihi.org.
16 Langley G, Nolan K, Nolan T, *et al. The Improvement Guide: a practical approach to enhancing organisational performance.* San Francisco: Jossey Bass Publishers; 1996.
17 NHS Institute for Innovation and Improvement. http://www.institute.nhs.uk/.

18 http://www.cchsa.ca/upload/files/pdf/ISQua/Introduction.pdf.

19 Middleton S, Roberts A. *Integrated Care Pathways: a practical approach to implementation.* London: Butterworth-Heinemann; 2000.

20 De Luc K. *Developing Care Pathways – the tool kit.* Oxford: Radcliffe Medical Press; 2001.

21 http://www.library.nhs.uk/pathways.

22 McDonald P, Whittle C, Dunn L, *et al.* Shortfalls in integrated care pathways: part 1: what don't they contain? *J Integ Care Pathways.* 2006; **10**(1): 17–22.

23 Mosher C, Cronk P, Kidd A, et *al.* Upgrading practice with critical pathways. *Am J Nurs* 1992; **1**: 41–4.

24 The National Assembly of Wales. *An introduction to Clinical Pathways, putting patients first.* Cardiff: HMSO; 1999.

25 Stead L, Arthur C, Cleary A. Do multi-disciplinary pathways of care affect patient satisfaction? *Health Care Risk Report.* 1995; **Nov**: 13–5.

26 Trubo R. If this is cookbook medicine, you may like it. *Medical Economics* 1993; **69**: 69–82.

27 www.mapofmedicine.com.

28 Currie L, Harvey G. *The origins and use of care pathways in the USA, Australia and the United Kingdom.* Report 15. Oxford: Royal College of Nursing Institute; 1998.

29 The Centre for Change and Innovation. www.cci.scot.nhs.uk.

Further reading

- Zander K. Integrated Care Pathways: eleven international trends. *J Integ Care Pathways* 2002; **6**:101–7.

- Harkleroad A, Schirf D, Volpe J, *et al.* Critical pathway development: An integrative literature review. *Am J Occup Ther.* 2000; **54**(2): 148–54.

- Chartered Society of Physiotherapy. *Integrated Care Pathways.* PA46. London: CSP; 2002.

- Trowbridge R, Weingarten S. *Making health care safer, a critical analysis of patient safety practices.* Chapter 52: Critical Pathways. Agency for Healthcare Research and Quality, 2001. http://www.ahrq.gov/clinic/ptsafety/chap52.htm.

- Van Herck P, Vanhaecht K, Sermeus W. Effects of Clinical Pathways: do they work? *J Integ Care Pathways* 2004; **8**: 95–105.

- http://www.18weeks.nhs.uk/public/default.aspx?load=ArticleViewer&ArticleId=645.

Chapter 4

Communication and the health professional

Anne Mandy and Gail Louw

Introduction

Good communication skills are essential for all health professionals. The fundamental problem about defining communication as nothing more than information exchange is that it is only a necessary, but not a sufficient, condition for understanding the complex process of communication.

What is communication?

Communication can be defined as 'the process by which information meanings and feelings are shared by people through the exchange of verbal and non-verbal messages'.[1] Communication is transmitted by speech, signals and writing, or through behavioural information such as thoughts and emotions in order that it can be satisfactorily received and understood. Understanding the meaning of the communication involves the process of contextualisation and is often referred to as the process of 'sharing meaning'. Communication could therefore be defined as: 'the management of messages for the purpose of creating meaning'. Therefore the goal of effective communication is the successful sharing of meaning. In order to be successful in creating meaning an understanding of the goals of communication is necessary. There are at least three general types of communication goals which are closely linked to the affective elements of communication. Self Presentation Goals reflect who we are and how we want to be perceived; Relational Goals reflect how we develop, maintain, and terminate relationships and Instrumental Goals which reflect how we manipulate others, gain compliance, manage interpersonal conflict, use and recognise interpersonal influence strategies. These goals are important and clearly influential in organisational communication.

Non-verbal communication

When individuals speak, they normally do not confine themselves to the mere emission of words. A great deal of meaning is conveyed by non-verbal means which always accompany oral discourse – intended or not. In other words, a spoken message is always sent on two levels simultaneously, verbal and non-verbal. Non-verbal communication consists of all the messages other than words that are used in communication. These symbolic messages are transferred by means of intonation, vocally produced noises, body posture, body gestures, facial expressions or pauses.

Non-verbal behaviour pre-dates verbal communication because from birth individuals can only use non-verbal means to express themselves. This innate character of non-verbal behaviour is important in communication. Even before a sentence is uttered, the hearer observes the body gestures and facial expressions of the speaker and uses these cues to try to make sense of the symbolic messages. They are perceived as trustworthy because they are usually unconscious and part of everyday behaviour. Thus it is assumed that non-verbal cues do not lie. However, respondents feel uncomfortable when the non-verbal message does not support the verbal message or at worst contradicts it. Conflict arises when the sense of non-verbal behaviour does not match the meaning of the communication. In such situations clarification is sought in order that the verbal message can be understood.

Non-verbal communication can be used to persuade or to control others, to clarify or embellish things, to stress, complement, regulate and repeat verbal expressions. They can also be used to substitute verbal expression, as this is the case with several body gestures. Non-verbal communication is emotionally expressive and so any discourse appealing to the receiver's emotions will have a persuasive impact.

An important additional component in health communication is touch of which two types can be distinguished. Functional touch is where health professionals make physical contact with a patient to aid diagnosis or to carry a specific procedure or therapeutic task. The other type of touch is therapeutic touch where body contact is used to comfort or console a patient. Similarly the form of touch employed is important in relation to compliance and adherence to treatment regimes.[2] There is a developing literature which explores the value of therapeutic touch.[3, 4, 5, 6, 7, 8, 9, 10, 11] Moreover, Dickson et al[12] review the components of non-verbal skills in detail for the health professional.

Clinical communication

Communication is a core clinical skill essential to clinical competence.[13] The fundamental components of communication have been described by several authors.[12,13,14] Similarly effective attributes have been described and key attributes identified to ensure effective health communication, which have given rise to the production of policy documentation.[15] There is also an extensive literature exploring the deficiencies that occur in professional communication and the subsequent consequences of poor communication.[16]

Other authors have considered in detail the components of communication including non-verbal behaviours[17] and listening and attending skills.[18] In light of this wealth of extensive literature, the fundamentals of communication will not be considered here. It is acknowledged that healthcare professionals communicate with all levels of employees. Dickson et al[12] identify ten groups of people with whom health professionals communicate: these include patient/client interactions, patient/client's relations, team communication, communication with other healthcare professionals, support staff, administrators, public, media, students and company representatives. Communication occurring in this type of environment can be described as organisational communication.

Organisational communication

Organisational communication occurs within a particular social system composed of interdependent groups attempting to achieve commonly recognised goals.

Organisational communication can include, for example the characteristics shown in Table 4.1:

Table 4.1 Characteristics of organisational communication.

Flow and direction of communication	This may be formal, informal, internal, external, upward, downward, horizontal or with networks
Induction procedures	Including new staff orientation procedures, policies and procedures and employee benefits
Channels of communication	Including electronic media such as e-mail, intranet, internet, teleconference, print media such as bullet boards, newsletters and face to face
Meetings	Briefings, staff meetings, project meetings, team meetings, finance meetings, commissioning meetings, Board meetings
Interviews	Selection, performance reviews, career development, discipline, grievance, competency

More recently, the field of organisational communication has moved from acceptance of more traditional mechanistic models such as information moving from a sender to a receiver, to a less hegemonic approach in which communication is used to accomplish certain tasks within an organisational setting and also to explore the impact of the organisation on staff.

Organisational communication can therefore be defined as that which occurs within a particular social system and is composed of interdependent groups attempting to achieve commonly recognised goals. The literature supports varied theories which explain the communication strategies which occur in organisations. One example is the Organisational Assimilation Theory described by Jablin.[19] This theory explains how new employees to an organisation assimilate into the organisation by using communication. Jablin[19] describes three stages that occur as one enters an organisation as Anticipatory Socialisation, Encounter Stage, and Metamorphosis. An individual's socialisation into an organisation determines his/her success within the organisation.

Alternatively there is Critical Theory which was proposed by Deetz.[20] The goal of this model is for employees to define their roles within the organisation. Such goals increase the feeling of being valued among employees, that they have a stake in the company. If more organisations took a critical approach there would be a greater likelihood of job satisfaction. The goal is to make the work place more cohesive, and to develop mutual understanding about an organisation's goals. Rather than having a traditional bureaucracy, the organisation should seek to improve its relations with the individuals that actually do the work.

Communication competence

Communication competence is the ability to choose a communication behaviour that is both appropriate and effective for a given situation. Interpersonal competency allows communication goals to be achieved without causing the other party to lose face. A commonly used model to describe competence is the component model[21] which includes three components: knowledge, skill, and motivation.

- Knowledge simply means adoption of the most appropriate behaviour in a given situation.
- Skill is having the ability to apply that behaviour.
- Motivation is wanting to communicate in a competent manner.

Communication competence is also dependent on the context in which the interaction takes place.[22, 23]

The component model asserts that communication competence is mutually defined by the interdependency of the cognitive component, the behavioural component and the affective component by the communicant in an interpersonal encounter. Rubin[23] explains that communication competence is:

an impression formed about the appropriateness of another's communicative behaviour and that one goal of the communication scholar is to understand how impressions about communication competence are formed, and to determine how knowledge, skill and motivation lead to perceptions of competence within various contexts.

Canary and Cody[24] provide six criteria for assessing competence:

1 adaptability
2 conversational involvement
3 conversational management
4 empathy
5 effectiveness
6 appropriateness.

1 Adaptability (flexibility)
The ability to change behaviours and goals to meet the needs of the interaction including:
- social experience – the ability to participate in various social interactions
- social composure – the ability to keep calm through accurate perception and interpretation of meaning of the communication
- social confirmation – the ability to acknowledge your partner's goals
- appropriate disclosure – the ability to be sensitive to the amount and type of information being disclosed
- articulation – the ability to express ideas through the use of appropriate language

- wit – the ability to use appropriate humour in adapting to social situations to ease tensions.

2 **Conversational involvement**
- Responsiveness – knowing what to say, understand the roles, interact appropriately.
- Perceptiveness – be aware of how others perceive you.
- Attentiveness – listen, don't be pre-occupied.

3 **Conversational management**
- How the interaction is regulated.
- Adaptation and control of social situations.
- Who controls the ebb and flow of the interaction and how smoothly the interaction proceeds.
- How topics proceed and change.

4 **Empathy**
- The ability to demonstrate understanding and share emotional reactions to the situation.
- Cognitive understanding.
- Parallel emotions.

5 **Effectiveness**
- Achieving the objectives of the conversation.
- Achieving personal goals.
- A fundamental criteria for determining competence.

6 **Appropriateness**
- Upholding the expectations for a given situation.
- A fundamental criteria for determining competence.

The significance of communication competence should not be underestimated. The way in which it is understood and defined will determine the approach adopted in training and evaluating healthcare communication interactions.

The concepts of communication, characteristics, skills, communication competencies have been described and explored. The characteristics and behaviours of team communication are now considered.

Team communication

Communication within teams is fundamental to effective healthcare practice. Team communication not only occurs transversely across teams, but also hierarchically with managers. Team communication is often a forum which is considered to be problematic and an area where potentially barriers can exist. Barriers often develop as a result of conflict stemming from deep seated social and professional differences. They tend to arise from different knowledge bases, methods of education, including rituals of socialisation and enculturation, and training 'tribalisms'.[25] Different professions have their own distinct occupational cultures and these may lead to distinct and identifiable groupings. Each professional group develops its own characteristic style of communication and language, which in turn leads to stereotypical judgements. Mandy et al[26] suggest that the way in which a profession is judged can in part be attributed to the nature of the practise. Their research explored stereotypical attitudes of undergraduate physiotherapy and podiatry students who were experiencing inter-professional education. The results suggested that physiotherapy students judged podiatry to be a more 'lowly' profession because it deals only with feet. Physiotherapy, however, may be ranked more highly because it has more glamorous connotations, for example being linked with sport and sporting heroes. They also suggested that such stereotypes may be manifestations of much more powerful archetypes. Archetypes are described as 'biological norms of psychic activity'[26] that exert an influence on experience which tends to then be organised according to a pre-existing pattern. 'Tribal' behaviours include intra-professional defences, other professionals being identified as wrong or different. Tribal characteristics can be divided into five categories:

1 language or dialect differences
2 thinking differences
3 value differences
4 training differences
5 rules that govern behavioural norms.

Bridging such gaps requires an understanding of such differences, and the development of professional respect. Linking the 'tribes' together through collaborative negotiation will reduce tribal behaviours.

This has important implications for team communication particularly where the team leader may be from a different discipline to professions within the team, as is often the case in the management of AHPs where a manager from one profession holds management responsibility for several AHP professions. The power and status accorded to professional groups can impinge on the way in which a multi-professional team operates and the behaviours that a team may exhibit. The way in which communication occurs and context in which it happens are both important factors to enable effective communication to take place. Furthermore individual philosophies of the meaning of effective communication and also an understanding of others' roles and how the role is valued are pivotal to successful communication.[27] Miller et al[27] identified three different philosophies held by different team members in their study.

1 The directive philosophy was based on an assumption of a hierarchy within the team in which one person would take the lead as a result of their status and power. This philosophy was most frequently held by members of the medical profession and some non-specialist nurses. The team leader would determine what, when and how information was communicated and to whom.
2 In the AHPs, social work professions, some health visitors and nurses, an integrative philosophy was observed. This philosophy acknowledged the complexity of communication and supported the belief that in-depth discussion and negotiation were important to be able to develop a team understanding of patients' needs. These groups recognised the importance of understanding the different contributions different professions provided and that each professional's contribution was of equal value.
3 The third type of philosophy discussed was the elective philosophy. This philosophy was held predominantly by professions that worked autonomously and referred to other professions when necessary. The communication style endorsed by such professionals demonstrated brevity seeking only to inform and there was an acknowledgement of a hierarchical structure of professional groups.

Parallel working can also occur within dysfunctional teams, where professionals accept that they need to liaise with other professions but only have a limited understanding of their respective roles. Adoption of such attitudes acknowledges the existence of hierarchical frameworks within teams and also within professions and is largely framed by beliefs in the medical model. It is assumed that powerful professions will be the decision makers and all other team members acquiesce or support those in powerful positions. In such instances communication is usually directive and brief. Sharing of knowledge and skills remains within professional boundaries.

In addition to these styles there is also formal and informal communication that occurs in various forums. Some of the most useful communication often takes place in informal settings. Corridor communication can be exclusive, targeted and extremely informative. Informal lunchtime discussions not only encourage the use of open and free discussions but can gain insight into who is invited and the possible power bases that exist. Conversely formal meetings may openly provide a forum in which to share information but can be hierarchical and may not provide the opportunity for open discussion and sharing of ideas. Communication in this case may involve coded 'management speak'.

Communication at different levels

Following the 1997 General Election there was, for a few years, a move away from 'customers and competition' to a greater emphasis on partnership, regulation and user involvement.[28] The 1999 Health Act[29] resulted in a framework of integrated health in which there was a 'duty of partnership' and a need for professionals to work together. The emphasis shifted towards service improvement and the commissioning of services. This impacted on communication through clinical governance initiatives which embodied the importance of addressing barriers between managers and doctors, and managers and health professionals.[30] A commonly identified barrier is lack of general understanding of each others' roles, each having their own agenda. Professional and managerial language and jargon may be perceived as exclusive resulting in a reduction of communication and integration leading to isolation. Owen[31] suggests that a strategy for successful working relationships to address this issue is for managers and clinicians to work and learn together at early stages of their careers where there is more likely to be greater flexibility and co-operation.

Newly promoted middle managers commonly concentrate on managing the people who report to them and sometimes forget about communicating with and managing the person to whom they report. Communicating across management strata effectively requires an understanding of certain factors and skills. Gabarro and Kotter[32] suggest that there is a 'mutually dependent relationship between two fallible human beings' in which the line manager is probably more dependent. An understanding of how the junior manager works will also facilitate the mechanism of communication to be adopted by the middle manager.

A manager who enjoys talking will respond more favourably to someone who is a patient listener. The careful selection of strategic questions is of paramount importance. Questions that ask their opinion are often welcomed such as; 'What do you think?' or 'How would you handle this?' If however, the manager prefers written communication the use of e-mails, notes or briefing papers may be more successful.

The managers' personality will also affect the style of communication that should be adopted. People who prefer formal relationships are often rigid, rule orientated and adopt policy procedures. These approaches are hierarchical, authoritarian and suggest that the manager requires a maximum amount of control. Surprises and deviations from plans are not readily acceptable. Conversely managers that prefer informality are often more flexible, trusting, and collegial. Introvert people must be drawn out whilst extrovert people will be more participative.

The decision making style of the manager is also an important consideration and will impact on the quality of the communication. Managers who are primarily judgmental will tend to see arguments in black-and-white. However, managers who have more perception may be more creative, intuitive and tend to see all sides of an argument and consequently may make a more balanced decision. It is also important to develop an understanding of behavioural style which will impact on communication. Behavioural style is a combination of interpersonal behaviours which focuses on how a person acts, speaks and the behaviours they adopt. It is suggested that there are four behavioural styles, discussed below.

It is also important to understand managers' corporate goals, expectations and priorities in order that all communication can be put in a context of helping the manager to achieve his/her goals. This enables the staff member to reach a mutual agreement with their manager about expectations – not only what he/she expects from them, but also what they expect from the job.

Effective and open channels of communication are also imperative. This is particularly important with managers who are keen to delegate. The amount and style of communication depends on the manager – as well as the content of the work – but as a middle manager it is imperative to understand the information needs of the junior managers and to learn how to manage them accordingly. Finally it is imperative to adopt an efficient use of the junior managers' time.

Concept of behavioural style

Behavioural style reflects a pervasive and enduring set of interpersonal behaviours which focuses on how a person acts rather than on what is said. A common model used throughout the centuries has focused on grouping human interactive behaviour into four categories. These categories typically represent quadrants along two dimensions of human behaviour.

Interactive dimensions

Merrill and Reid[33] suggest that there are two dimensions of interpersonal behaviour, which include assertiveness and responsiveness. Assertiveness is perceived as the degree to which others see behaviours being enforced or driven. Responsiveness is the degree to which behaviours are seen as emotionally expressive or emotionally controlled. Behavioural style is determined almost exclusively through interpretation of what is observed from human interactions.

Four basic behavioural styles

A person's behavioural style exists from childhood and is a function of both heredity and environment. Each person has a dominant behavioural style that is reflected in how that individual works, interacts and communicates with others. This behavioural style is readily observed by others, but is often difficult to identify correctly in oneself. Therefore, the development of observation skills and the application of these to an individual is the key to understanding a person's behavioural style. Similarly the best way to identify one's own behavioural style is to receive knowledgeable and insightful feedback from others.

Bolton and Bolton[34] suggest that there are four categories of behavioural style described in Box 4.1.

1 The analyser
2 The director
3 The socialiser
4 The relater

Box 4.1 Categories of behavioural style.

- **The analyser – the thought person**
  This behavioural style incorporates a low level of assertiveness and a low level of responsiveness. Analysers exhibit behaviours which are precise, deliberate and systematic. They assimilate and process information without emotion. Such an approach results in information being gathered and evaluated prior to it being articulated or actioned. Such people are generally industrious, objective and well-organised but rarely combine work with friendship or express feelings of warmth. In addition analysers exhibit traits of self-control and caution and are considered to be people who prefer analytical justification to emotional claims. As a result of this they are often viewed as being a bit formal and tend to resist compromise in problem situations.

- **The director – the action person**
  This style combines a low level of emotional responsiveness with a relatively high degree of assertiveness. Such individuals tend to be task-oriented, are focused, able to express themselves succinctly, and get to the point quickly. Directors are independent and demonstrate behaviours that are often pragmatic, results-oriented, objective and competitive. They are achievers and are commonly found in positions of authority and are central to decision-making processes in organisations. Directors are firm and forceful people, they are confident, decisive and generally risk-takers in interactive situations. Such traits are often perceived as concerning for colleagues which in turn can result in conflict. Moreover, the directors leave little doubt about who is in charge of an issue that is being considered.

- **The socialiser – the front man**
  This behavioural style integrates high levels of both emotional responsiveness and assertiveness. Such people are creative and inspirational and are able to take an overview from a different perspective. They employ novel and creative approaches to problems and are willing to take risks in order to seize opportunities, particularly in interactive situations. They therefore act quickly and make instant

decisions. They have a developed ability to charm, persuade, enthuse and motivate people and can be a strong motivating force. They may be perceived as radical, extrovert and over zealous to more cautious colleagues. This type of individual is extrovert, optimistic and enthusiastic who likes to be at the centre of attention and is a whirlwind of ideas.

- **The relater – the people person**
  This behavioural style demonstrates above average responsiveness with comparatively low level assertiveness. Such individuals are sympathetic and sensitive to the needs of others. Their altruistic qualities enable them to understand others more deeply. They employ the skills of empathy and understanding in interpersonal problem-solving situations. They are trusting and trustworthy which enables them to bring out the best in their colleagues. Relaters are team players who like stability and who care greatly about relationships with others. They are amiable, often somewhat timid and slow to change and generally resist direct confrontational involvement.

Strengths and weaknesses of each style

The strengths and weaknesses of each behavioural style are summarised and shown in Figure 4.1. Usually an individual lacks the strengths of the style diagonally across the grid from his or her own style. An effective leadership team is composed of individuals from each of the quadrants in the table.

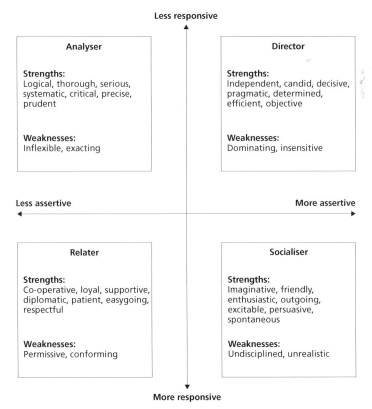

Figure 4.1 The strengths and weaknesses of each behavioural style adapted from Bolton and Bolton.[34]

The behavioural style paradigm is an important reference point for evaluating team dynamics. The best and most productive interpersonal relationships and communications occur when two styles become complementary with each individual's strengths, thereby compensating for the weaknesses of the other.

Styles within teams and organisations

The functional dynamics of a team are greatly affected by the styles of its members[35] which in turn will impact directly on leadership. Leadership tasks require a combination of all four behavioural types in a manager.[36] Drucker also suggests that finding the strengths of all four types in one person is virtually impossible. The most productive teams do however, exhibit a balance of each of the behavioural styles amongst the team members. This gives rise to teams which will be more cohesive and able to work together for the benefit of the organisation. Moreover an understanding of the behavioural style paradigm of all those involved assists with this interaction and facilitates a greater respect for the diversity within the group.

Communication styles of each category

The preferred communication style of each category is shown in Table 4.2.

- **The analyser** – analysers prefer logical systematic conversations, not spontaneous impromptu reactions. They have a good attention span and are good listeners. They are usually the conservative members of the organisation.
- **The director** – action orientated directors have short attention spans, interrupt conversations and avoid small talk. They have a pragmatic approach, are efficient and objective. Meetings are ideally short and to the point. The directors are the doers of the organisation.
- **The relater** – typically interested in others' lives, sensitive to moods and feelings and would prefer to interact in social settings. Their offices will include comfortable chairs in which to sit and chat with tea and coffee making facilities. They are often considered the conscience of an organisation. They feel uncomfortable with behaviours that fail to take into consideration human elements.
- **The socialiser** – enthusiastic, imaginative, ideas people who may not have highly developed interpersonal skills. Their passion can sometimes make people feel uncomfortable in their presence and can be perceived as potentially volatile members.

For communication to be effective and productive a combination of interpersonal relationships is desirable whereby the styles are complementary. The strengths of each can then be maximised and used to the benefit of the other party. When behavioural styles and communication abilities are understood a synergistic relationship will develop.

This section has explored communication in relation to behavioural styles and identified the preferred communication media for each style. In the next section electronic communication is reviewed in relation to healthcare management.

Table 4.2 Communication styles, limitations and most preferred electronic communication style.

Behavioural style	Preferred communication style	Personal limitations in communication	Preferred media
Analyser	Direct, formal, efficient economical. Meetings controlled by an agenda and minuted.	Inability to make use of flexible working. Unable to take advantage of informal networks, for example corridor conversations.	Formal e-mail. Formal telephone conversations.
Director	Adopt formal communication styles for formal and informal settings. Formal short meetings. Formal letters or memoranda.	Would not like others to alter or amend their contribution (for example Wikis). Not being in control. Would not like free communication. Would not allow digression or 'non-relevant contributions'	Formal e-mail. Telephone.
Relater	Informal. Opportunistic conversations (whether appropriate or not).	Not always able to adopt the most appropriate manner and behaviour in a specific forum, for example being flippant or humorous in formal meetings.	Informal e-mail. Telephone. Blogs. Wikis. Video/ teleconferences.
Socialiser	Informal. Opportunistic conversations (usually has social skills to assess appropriateness). Allows others to express themselves.	Keeping quiet. Allowing silences. Disciplined delivery of information.	E-mail. Wikis. Blogs. Telephone.

Electronic communication and healthcare management

The basis of communication in management has been shown to be different from the type of communication and skills required in the clinical situation. Communication in management has further been affected by the impact of electronic communication which has pervaded healthcare over the past decade. Electronic communication has insidiously grown and developed and has afforded ease and speed of communication institutionally, nationally and internationally.

As with any means of communication, it has rules and applications which may be formal or informal.

There are many types of electronic communication, but the ones that are perhaps the most important and most widely used in healthcare communication are e-mail, blogs and wikis. E-mail is perhaps the most commonly used form, is particularly useful and will be discussed in greater detail than the others.

E-mail communication

E-mail was first developed in 1971, by an engineer Ray Tomlinson assigned to a project called send message (SNDMSG). This program was not new; it had existed for a number of years. By today's standards it was primitive. All it did was allow users on the same machine to send messages to each other. Users could create text files which would then be delivered to mailboxes on the same machine. Over the past 30 years it has evolved and developed and is now the most commonly used electronic communication tool.

Over the last 35 years electronic communication has become increasingly important which in turn has resulted in new demands being placed upon language and variations in written language.[37] Furthermore the rules governing language use have changed as a result of the electronic medium. The language used in electronic communication is either formal or informal. Informal language contains text based icons and acronyms for managing social interactions and changes to spelling norms and in addition the electronic medium provides a new context for the writing process.

Word processing and the flexible nature of electronic text has resulted in thoughts being committed to writing far more quickly than when it was necessary to rely on paper and pens. Furthermore it is easy to make changes on the electronic screen[38] to edit and modify. Within the informal style of e-mail, users are able to be creative with presentation, improvisation and involve the use of humour. Trupe[39] observed multiple writer identities through the use of a range of linguistic techniques including range of word choice and syntax. Such elements of electronic communication form part of an emergent cultural diversity. The luxury of creativity and informality within this form of communication can however, result in tension when inappropriately used. The traditional norms governing the language and presentation of official letters and documents are clearly different to the rules of e-mail.

One of the fundamental differences between e-mail communication and verbal communication is the lack of non-verbal and visual cues provided in an oral discourse. Caution is urged when including humour in e-mail which may be misunderstood. Visual cues of paralanguage, kinesics and synchrony to complement verbal language are unavailable to 'on line' writers. However, these cues can be articulated through e-mail using text based emoticons, punctuation and politeness markers.

Conversely the lack of visual cues can be used to an advantage particularly as it reduces the intimidation factor.[38] Some people prefer the neutrality and anonymity of e-mail.

The use of e-mail as means of communication in management is an important issue. Panici[40] describes technological literacy as 'understanding both the why and how of new media communication tools'. This goes beyond pure technological skills, which are relatively easy to obtain, to encompass critical thinking skills and key issues surrounding the new technology issues such as privacy, intellectual property and assessing source reliability.

Blogs

A blog is a website where entries are made in journal style and displayed in a reverse chronological order. They have a simple structure, are generally personal although they can be used by a group and allow comments to be added. The term blog was first defined by Jorn Barger in 1997 as 'a web page where a Web logger "logs" all the other pages she finds interesting'.[41] Blogging has rapidly gained in popularity. The site Xanga was launched in 1996 and had only 100 entries by 1997. However, by December 2005 it had over two million entries.

Bloggers are driven to document their lives, provide commentary and opinion, express deeply felt emotions, articulate ideas through writing and form and maintain community forums.

Wikis

Wikis are documents that are open for all members within a group or organisation to access. It is a group communication mechanism whereby members of the group are allowed to contribute to the discussion, to make changes to their input and to edit contributions already made by others. Every contributor has equal rights and can participate.

Wikis are potentially useful devices for organisations to capture the learning within their workplace. Previous problems associated with employees leaving and taking with them the learning they may have accumulated over years, leaving a gap within the organisation, may well be overcome by this ongoing device. The first ever wikis site was created for the Portland Pattern Repository in 1995. That site now hosts tens of thousands of pages.

Conclusion

The art of communication in healthcare and healthcare management has clearly changed and developed over the past few years. Successful team management includes an understanding of behavioural styles of staff members and using this to unite people with complementary styles cohesively. This in turn enables a team to develop synergy. Moreover, an innovative use of appropriate electronic communication will enhance team working and facilitate communication in an economic and efficient way.

References

1 Brooks W, Heath R. *Speech communication*. Dubuque, Iowa: W.C Brown: 1985.
2 Peters R. The effectiveness of therapeutic touch: a meta-analytic review. *Nurs Sci Q.* 1999; **12**: 52–61.
3 Gagne D, Toye R. The effects of therapeutic touch and relaxation therapy in reducing anxiety. *Arch Psych Nurs.* 1994; **8**: 184–9.

4 Keller E, Bzdek V. Effects of therapeutic touch on tension headache pain. *Nurs Res.* 1986; **35**: 101–6.

5 Meehan T. Therapeutic touch and postoperative pain: a Rogerian research study. *Nurs Sci Q.* 1993; **6**: 69–78.

6 Wirth D. Complementary healing intervention and dermal wound reepithelialization: an overview. *Int J Psychosom.* 1995; **42**: 48–53.

7 Turner J, Clark A, Gauthier D. The effect of therapeutic touch on pain and anxiety in burn patients. *J Adv Nurs.* 1998; **28**: 10–20.

8 Gordon A, Merenstein J, D'Amico F. The effects of therapeutic touch on patients with osteoarthritis of the knee. *J Fam Pract.* 1998; **47**: 271–7.

9 Ireland M. Therapeutic touch with HIV-infected children: a pilot study. *J Assoc Nurs AIDS Care.* 1998; **9**: 68–77.

10 Quinn J. Therapeutic touch as energy exchange: replication and extension. *Nurs Sci Q.* 1989; **2**: 79–87.

11 Rosa L, Rosa E, Sarner L. A close look at therapeutic touch. *JAMA.* 1998; **279**: 1005–10.

12 Dickson D, Hargie O, Morrow N. *Communication Skills Training for Health Professionals.* 2nd ed. Cheltenham: Nelson Thornes; 2003.

13 Kurtz S, Silverman J, Draper J. *Teaching and learning Communication Skills in Medicine.* Oxford: Radcliffe; 2005.

14 Ley P. *Communicating with Patients: improving communication, satisfaction and compliance.* London: Chapman and Hall; 1988.

15 http://www.healthypeople.gov.

16 Davis H, Fallowfield L. *Counselling and Communication in Healthcare.* Chichester: Wiley; 1991.

17 Argyle M. *The Psychology of Interpersonal Behaviour.* Harmondsworth: Penguin; 1972.

18 Morrison P, Burnard P. *The Interpersonal Relationship in Nursing.* 2nd ed. Basingstoke: Macmillan; 1997.

19 Jablin F. Organizational communication: an assimilation approach. In: Roloff M, Berger C, editors. *Social Cognition and Communication.* Sage; 1982: 255–86.

20 Deetz S. Critical interpretive research in organizational communication. *Western J Speech Comm.* 1982; **46**: 131–49.

21 Spitzberg B, Cupach W. *Interpersonal Communication Competence.* Beverly Hills, CA: Sage; 1984.

22 Cody M, McLaughlin M. The situation as a construct in interpersonal communication research. In: McLaughlin ML, Miller GR, editors. *Handbook of Interpersonal Communication.* Beverly Hills, CA: Sage; 1985.

23 Rubin R. The validity of the communication competency assessment instrument. *Communication Monographs.*1985; **52**: 173–85.

24 Canary D, Cody M, Manusov V, editors. *Interpersonal communication: a goals-based approach.* NY: Bedford St. Martin's; 2003.

25 Atkins J. Triablism, Loss and Grief: issues for multiprofessional education. *J Interprof Care.* 1998; **12**: 303–7.

26 Mandy A, Milton C, Mandy P. Professional stereotyping and interprofessional education. *Learning in Health and Social Care.* 2004; **3**(3): 154–70.

27 Miller C, Freedman M, Ross N. *Interprofessional Practice in Health and Social Care. Challenging the shared learning agenda.* Arnold Publishers: London; 2001.

28 Barnes M. Users as citizens: collective action and the local governance of welfare. *Social Policy and Administration.* 1999; **33**(1): 73–90.

29 Health Act. 1999. Available at: http://www.opsi.gov.uk/.

30 Headrick L, Wilcock P, Batalden P. Interprofessional working and continuing medical education. *BMJ.* 1998; **316**: 771–4.

31 Owen J, Phillips K. Ignorance is not bliss. Doctors, managers and development. *J Manag Med.* 2000; **14**(2): 119–29.

32 Gabarro J, Kotter J. Managing your boss. *Harvard Business Review*. 1993; **71**(1): 150–8.

33 Merrill D, Reid R. *Personal Styles and Effective Performance*. Radnor, PA: Chilton; 1981.

34 Bolton R, Bolton D. Social Style/Management Style. New York; American Management Association: 1984.

35 Hambrick D, Mason P. Upper echelons: the organization as a reflection of its top managers. *Acad Manage Rev*. 1984; **9**(2): 193–206.

36 Drucker P. *Management: tasks, responsibilities, and practices*. New York: Harper & Row; 1973.

37 Biesenbach-Lucas S, Wiesenforth D. Email and word processing in the ESL classroom: how the medium affects the message. *Lang Learn Technol*. 2001; **5**(1): 39–53.

38 Leibowitz W. Technology transforms writing and the teaching of writing. *Chronicle of Higher Education*. 1999; **46** (14): A67–A68.

39 Trupe A. Academic Literacy in a Wired World: redefining genres for college. Available at: http://english.ttu.edu/kairos/7.2/sectionone/trupe/WiredWorld.htm.

40 Panici D. New media and the introductory mass communication course. *Journalism Mass Comm Educator*. 1998; **53**(1), 52–63.

41 Blood R. Weblogs: a history and perspective. Rebecca's Pocket: 2000. www.rebeccablood.net/essays/weblog_history.html.

Chapter 5

Managing staff and Human Resources

Helen Anderson

Introduction

The challenge in managing staff and human resources is making an organisation or team, however large or small, a place where people want to give of their best and do highest quality work.

Previously Human Resource Management (HRM) was about managing a resource, today it is seen in the more modern context of people being a major source of competitive advantage. Within healthcare that means using every opportunity available to foster an environment where staff individual and team levels are motivated to provide excellent patient care. With greater resources being allocated to healthcare the demand from patients and government for continually increasing improvements in standards of patient care, patient outcomes and value for money is relentless.

Modern HRM practice at a strategic level ensures that the people dimension is integral to organisational strategy. Emphasis is placed on the alignment of policies and practices such as:

- validated recruitment and selection methods
- learning and development programmes for all staff that lead to performance improvement
- effective performance appraisal schemes
- modern pay and reward systems
- encouraging more staff input at all levels into decision making
- more emphasis on team working
- attention to work/life balance issues
- valuing diversity and equality of opportunity.

Managers and leaders within the NHS are working within a more progressive HRM environment with the drive for modernisation through Agenda for Change (AfC) and Improving Working Lives (IWL). IWL aimed to support organisational culture change and embed good HRM practice at the heart of service delivery. This is driven, in part, by a body of research which shows that there is a positive correlation between effective people management practice and performance. Managing in ways that maximises benefits and outcomes *both for patients and staff* is at the core of a successful strategy.

This chapter focuses on three key areas that can make a significant contribution to good people management and effective performance:

1 understanding the environmental factors and managerial styles that create the circumstances in which people want to do excellent work and the crucial role of front line managers in bringing people management policies to life
2 developing the essential elements for effective team working and the evidence which points to improved outcomes for patients
3 the Investors in People (IIP) Standard as a benchmark to follow for learning and development and performance improvement.

Managers who are interested in finding out more about good people management and the drivers for effective performance can access a wide range of books and body of knowledge and research from professional bodies such as the Chartered Institute of Personnel and Development, Chartered Society of Physiotherapy and Business Schools of universities. Whilst much of this research is not health specific there is increasing interest in healthcare as an area for research. In addition articles in newspapers and publicity in the news media for initiatives such as the '100 Best Companies to Work For' also raise the profile of good people management and success through effective people management practices in the economy as a whole.

A basic starting point for managers is to understand the legal contract of employment between an employer and employee and the respective obligations of each of the parties. However the legal contract by itself is not sufficient to give managers enough information on what they can expect from their staff, how they can get the best from their staff and how they can nurture an environment in which the focus is on improved performance and better outcomes for patients. As far as the employee is concerned they will have contributed very little to the terms of the legal contract other than accepting them. In extreme cases the nature and content of the legal contract may only become clear when it is tested in an employment tribunal.

There have been significant shifts in thinking about what constitutes the essence of the modern employment relationship and the best ways for managers to encourage staff to work in innovative ways that will increase productivity generally. In healthcare improved standards of patient care and patient outcomes are key objectives for front line managers. As well as the legal contract of employment many managers believe the idea of a 'psychological contract' gives them a helpful framework to think about relationships at work. The psychological contract has been defined by Guest and Conway[1] as '... the perceptions of the two parties, employee and employer of what their mutual obligations are towards each other'. Some of these obligations will often be informal and imprecise others may be seen by employees as 'promises'. For example the 'promises' to provide staff with a career and a reasonably secure job, the expectation that there will be opportunities to develop and receive training and most importantly that their manager will treat them with fairness and respect. The key issue is that they are perceived by the employee to be part of the relationship with the employer. From a manager's perspective it is often the psychological contract that will be more influential than the legal contract in influencing how staff carry out their roles on a day-to-day basis.

Guest[1] has set out a useful model of the psychological contract which proposes that:

- the extent to which employers adopt people management practices will influence the state of the psychological contract
- the contract is based on employees' sense of fairness and trust and their belief that the employer is honouring the 'deal' between them
- where the psychological contract is positive, employee commitment and satisfaction will have a positive impact on business performance.

To get the best from their people organisations have to know what their employees expect from work. This has led to more and more emphasis on feedback and involvement via staff surveys, focus groups, 360 degree feedback and more involvement in decision making and upward communication. The IIP model has an explicit indicator that measures whether staff are encouraged to take ownership and responsibility by being involved in decision making.

Front line managers play a key role in ensuring that the psychological contract is healthy and productive. Whilst general policy and practice and communication from senior management can make some difference it is the quality of the relationship between individual managers and staff that has been shown to make a significant difference to how staff judge their organisations. By treating all their staff fairly, with respect and positively developing a relationship based on trust front line managers are best placed to influence employee commitment, satisfaction and performance.

What is the state of the psychological contract today?

Major national surveys between 1996 and 2004[2] show that:

- a majority of employees consistently report that they are satisfied with their jobs
- four out of five employees are not worried about losing their job and most expect that if they did lose their job they would be able to find another one at similar pay without having to move house
- levels of commitment have not shown any significant trend – whether up or down – in recent years
- trust in the organisation has declined particularly in the public sector
- there are widespread concerns about long hours and work intensity.

Whilst these surveys give managers a broad understanding of employees' views a deeper understanding of the specific ingredients of workplace environments that inspire people to want to give of their best and do excellent work can be found in the annual lists of organisations held up as the best in the country to work for, published by two national newspapers, the *Financial Times* and the *Sunday Times*.

Research published in Leary-Joyce[3] 'Becoming an Employer of Choice' based on the Sunday Times 100 Best Companies to Work For awards shows that if you want to become an employer of choice then you must fulfil the areas outlined in Box 5.1.

> **Box 5.1 Requirements of an employer of choice.**
>
> - Provide an environment in which colleagues can thrive and shine
> - Support and challenge staff to access the best in themselves
> - Set high standards and be rigorous in appraisal
> - Build strong relationships understanding the talents, strengths and needs of individual people
> - Acknowledge and celebrate success – make work a joy as well as a job
> - Build high trust throughout the organisation
> - Be a model in your own work; stretch yourself, live the organisation's principles, have fun, work hard and celebrate your success.

The challenge for managers within the AHPs is that many of the conditions for being an employer of choice as set out by Leary-Joyce are directly within their managerial control. For example:

- providing an environment in which colleagues can thrive and shine
  The AHPs provide interesting and demanding work for staff at all levels. Managers can play a significant role in creating the local environment in which their own staff can thrive and work to a level which makes a real difference to improved patient care and outcomes.
- support and challenge staff to access the best in themselves
  Within the NHS there is a greater emphasis on learning and development for all levels of staff. This needs to be supported by front line managers facilitating opportunities at team and individual levels for learning and development. This can be key in ensuring that managers are delivering on their side of the psychological contract.
- acknowledge and celebrate success – make work a joy as well as a job
  All managers can 'catch' staff doing things well and provide individual and team acknowledgement. Whilst recognition has long been a powerful motivator it is surprising how underused this basic technique is. Maslow's work on the hierarchy of needs[4] demonstrates that recognition is a key means of improving satisfaction and commitment.

Organisational issues that are not directly in the control of managers such as developing a rigorous appraisal system have been tackled as part of the reforms within AfC. The thrust of IWL, other retention and work/life balance initiatives and improvements in equality and diversity policy and practice all have a part to play in ensuring that organisationally people are treated fairly and building trust. However, the key role of the front line manager in treating staff fairly and building trust within their own teams cannot be overemphasised.

It is increasingly recognised that managers face a greater expansion of their roles with a greater recognition of the key contribution they make in bringing management policies and practices to life and their impact on the discretionary/citizenship behaviour of their staff. Increasing recognition is also being given to how managers can manage in a way which acknowledges that their staff can exercise significant choices about the pace at which they will work, how they will do their work and whether they will contribute to innovative ways of improving outcomes for patients.

Factors such as organisational restructuring and decline of middle managers, growth in team working, increasing recognition that responsibility for managing people rests with the line manager rather than a specialist and the move to leaner methods of working has increased the workload on front line managers. Front line managers have a key role to play in maintaining commitment, and surveys tell us[3] that employees tend to have more confidence in their line manager with whom they come into contact on a regular basis than in anonymous members of senior management.

The fact that trust in the organisation is declining in the public sector is a concern for managers and leaders and places a particular onus on front line managers to work at maintaining commitment and motivation. Research evidence[3] shows that where staff believe that management have not delivered or have broken promises or agreements then this has a negative effect on job satisfaction and commitment and on the psychological contract as a whole. It is particularly important therefore that front line managers follow through on any commitments they make to staff for example any learning and development opportunities they have promised to staff.

In this context equality and diversity considerations are particularly important. IWL accreditation requires NHS employers to demonstrate that they are investing in improving diversity and tackling discrimination and harassment. Managers will have a key role in playing their part in delivering on this agenda. IIP accreditation also has an explicit indicator that requires that strategies for managing people are designed to promote equality of opportunity in the development of the organisation's staff.

Team working

There is a large body of research on teams and team working. Recent research within the healthcare sector is particularly interesting in demonstrating a correlation between the management of staff and patient mortality in acute hospitals.

Katzenbach and Smith in 'The Wisdom of Teams'[5] and 'The Discipline of Teams'[6] define a team as:

> ... a small number of people with complementary skills who are committed to a common purpose, performance goals, and approach for which they hold themselves mutually accountable.

One of their fundamental beliefs is that 'a common performance objective is much more motivating for effective teams than the desire to be a team'. In defining objectives the difference between outcome based goals and activity based goals are highlighted. The authors state that people in most organisations chase after activity based goals or goals that describe the activities to be done instead of the performance impacts or outcomes those activities are supposed to produce. They also stress the importance of the group creating and managing itself according to a performance agenda.

Within the NHS great emphasis is increasingly placed on developing multidisciplinary and interdisciplinary team working. A major national study of team working in the NHS and the factors associated with it was done by the

Healthcare Team Effectiveness Project. This is a national study of team working in primary, secondary and community mental healthcare and research on team working in breast cancer care.[7] The model of team effectiveness[7] used considers the relationship between team inputs, processes and outputs as set out in Table 5.1.

Table 5.1 Model of team effectiveness. From Team Working and Effectiveness in Healthcare: Findings from the Healthcare Team Effectiveness Project.[7]

Team inputs: for example; size of team, the task, the diversity of the members' professional backgrounds.
Team processes: for example; information sharing, shared influence over decision-making, conflict management, clarifying objectives.
Team outputs: for example; number of patients seen, quality of care, innovation, team member satisfaction and stress.

Inputs	Team processes	Outputs
Domain	Leadership	Effectiveness – self and externally rated
Healthcare environment	Clarity of objectives	Clinical outcomes/quality of healthcare
Organisational context	Participation	
	Task orientation	Innovation – self and externally rated
Team task	Support for innovation	Cost-effectiveness
Team composition	Reflexivity	Team member mental health
	Decision making	Team member turnover
	Communication/integration	

This research shows the importance of team working in ensuring that health and social care are of the highest quality and efficiency. The conclusions were that:

- healthcare teams that have clear objectives, high levels of participation, emphasis on quality and support for innovation, provide high quality patient care. Such teams also introduce innovations in patient care
- members of teams that work well together have relatively low levels of stress
- in primary healthcare teams particularly – a diverse range of professional groups working together – is associated with higher levels of innovation in patient care
- the quality of meetings, communication and integration processes in healthcare teams, contributes to the introduction of new and improved ways of delivering patient care
- clear leadership contributes to effective team processes, to high quality patient care and to innovation.

The research showed that teams which worked well together provided support for each other during stressful or difficult times. It was also the case that staff who worked in teams perceived that there was more co-operation within the organisation than those who did not work in teams. This was a useful buffer against the negative effects of organisational issues that were perceived by others as stressful. It was also the case that the greater the proportion of managers in the team the lower stress levels amongst team members.

In primary healthcare those teams that had at least one meeting per week had introduced a greater number of, and more substantial innovations in, patient care than those that had fewer meetings.

In the research a minority, one third, of primary healthcare teams reported having a single clear leader. This lack of clear leadership was associated with lower levels of patient care and innovation. The research emphasised that there is a need to promote team leadership training within the NHS for those who are involved with leading or participating in teams. This supports the emerging work referred to earlier in the chapter on the importance of front line managers and their role in leading their teams and creating the environment in which their staff can thrive.

Two practical workbooks have been developed by Borrill and West[7,8] to assist in the implementation of team-working. They provide very useful audit tools to assess how well the organisation provides a context that is supportive to team working and how team leaders are carrying out their roles. They also provide practical advice and guidance for managers and team members on improving team working.

The guide for managers describes the role of the team leader as evolving into more of a facilitator/coach and creating an environment in which the benefits of team working are maximised and the weaknesses are minimised.

It states that team leadership can be the responsibility of one person or may be shared and that there are three complementary tasks to be carried out of leading, managing and coaching.

Box 5.2 Team leadership tasks.

- Leading the team:
  1 creating favourable performance conditions for the team
  2 building and maintaining the team as a performance unit
  3 coaching and supporting the team.
- Managing the team:
  1 setting clear, shared objectives
  2 clarifying the roles of team members
  3 developing individual tasks
  4 evaluating individual contributions
  5 providing feedback on team performance
  6 reviewing team processes, strategies and objectives.
- Coaching the team
  1 Listening
  2 Recognising and revealing feelings
  3 Giving feedback
  4 Agreeing goals

The guide for team members provides information about team working and the environment needed to promote effective team working. In particular it suggests that some of the key elements that influence whether a team will be effective other than the skills, knowledge and experience of individual team members are, see Box 5.3.

Box 5.3 Key elements to promote effective team working.

- Individuals feeling that they are important to the success of the team. Team members roles being developed in ways that make them indispensable and essential.
- The team as a whole having interesting tasks to perform.
- Individual contributions being identifiable and subject to evaluation. People not only feeling that their work is indispensable but also that other team members can see and acknowledge the contribution they make.
- Clear, shared team goals with built in performance feedback.
- An organisational context that supports team working.
- Effective team leadership.

The overall conclusion was that good teamwork makes a critical contribution to effectiveness and innovation in healthcare delivery and is good for the people who work in teams.

It also demonstrated that innovation and creativity could flourish where the environment and management make it safe to experiment. The level of trust built up within the team and with the team manager provides the foundation for innovations in patient care.

This research reinforces what has emerged from the work described earlier on the psychological contract and the environmental factors that lead staff to be willing to exercise their discretion about how they will do their work and whether they will contribute to innovative ways of improving outcomes for patients.

Recent research widely reported in the professional and national press by West et al [9] revealed strong associations between HRM practices and patient mortality generally. Three key HRM practices were identified that are likely to be associated with high levels of performance:

- appraisal
- identifying and meeting training needs and providing feedback to improve performance
- percentage of staff working in teams.

In terms of appraisal the research showed that the extent and sophistication of appraisal in the hospitals was particularly strongly related to patient mortality. Where the appraisal system provided for work objectives and training needs to be clearly identified and staff were given feedback to improve their performance there was a significant association with measures of patient mortality.

Interestingly the research suggested that it might be possible to influence hospital performance significantly by implementing sophisticated and extensive training and appraisal systems and encouraging a high percentage of employees to work in teams. Whilst the authors acknowledge that more research is needed to examine the underlying mechanisms responsible for the association it is certainly an important area for further research.

Investors in people

This chapter has focused on the environmental and managerial factors that create the circumstances in which people want to do great work, the crucial role of front line managers and the importance of team working. These are strong themes in IIP.

IIP is a benchmark learning and development standard which starts from the point that a strategy for improving the performance of the organisation is clearly articulated and understood at *all* levels of the organisation. It is a holistic framework to ensure that people have the right knowledge, skills and motivation to work efficiently. It aims to help organisations find the most suitable way to achieve success through their staff. There are currently over 37,000 recognised organisations in the UK employing over 27% of the UK workforce. It has been adopted by a number of units in the NHS and healthcare sector. Some of the practical benefits of working towards the standard include:

- customer satisfaction
- improved motivation
- public recognition
- enhanced quality.

Plan – developing strategies to improve the performance of the organisation (4 indicators)

Do – take action to improve the performance of the organisation (4 indicators)

Review – evaluating the impact of the performance of the organisation (2 indicators)

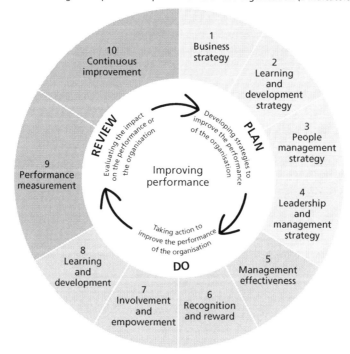

Figure 5.1 The three principles of IIP standards – reproduced with kind permission © Investors in People UK 2005 www.investorsinpeople.co.uk and www.investorsinpeople.co.uk/health.

There are three principles of the standard underpinned by 10 indicators as set out in Figure 5.1.[10]

Organisations compare their current practice against each indicator in the standard, assess gaps and implement an action plan. Whilst there is no typical time to achieve the standard it may be reasonable to expect that an organisation could achieve recognition within a year. Assessment includes site visits, where an assessor will discuss with a range of managers and staff what is happening in reality. As shown by the indicators below the evidence requirements are substantial.

Plan

Indicators 1–4   Developing Strategies to improve the performance of the organisation.

Indicator 1: a strategy for improving the performance of the organisation is clearly defined and understood.
This indicator sets the overall business framework. Experience has shown that most successful organisations have a strategy and business plan and set out clearly how they are going to improve their performance. The importance of staff understanding the purpose and vision of the organisation and how they personally contribute to success is key. It is expected that managers will actively seek the involvement of their staff in developing the business plan and in agreeing individual and team objectives.

An IIP assessor will expect staff to be able to explain the objectives of the organisation and their team, as well as their own objectives, at a level appropriate to their role. The healthcare effectiveness research shows that high levels of participation contribute to high quality patient care.

Where there are trades unions and representative groups they will be asked by the IIP assessor to confirm that top managers make sure that there are constructive relationships and that they are consulted when developing the organisation's business plan.

Indicator 2: learning and development is planned to achieve the organisation's objectives.
As shown by the IIP graphic, this is an holistic approach in which the strategic importance of learning and development and achieving organisational objectives is emphasised and linked to managers, teams and individual staff. Planning the resources necessary to fulfil the plans and how these link to clear objectives and outcomes are the fundamental building blocks.

It is focused on improved performance and outcomes and links back to Katzenbach's and Smith's[6] emphasis on outcome based goals and the performance impact from learning and development activities. This is not learning for learning's sake but steers organisations towards learning and development activities that will have an impact on specific objectives and performance.

An IIP assessor will ask a sample of managers to explain their team learning and development needs, what is planned to meet these needs, how these link to the achieving team and organisational objectives and their evaluation methods.

Staff will be asked by the assessor to outline how they have been involved in identifying their learning and development needs, how these will be met and what they hope to achieve at an individual, team and organisational level.

Indicator 3: strategies for managing people are designed to promote equality of opportunity in the development of the organisation's people.
IWL accreditation requires NHS employers to demonstrate that they are investing in improving diversity. This specific IIP indicator requires that equality of opportunity is built into the people management strategies.

At an individual level an assessor will ask staff if they believe that their manager is genuinely committed to making sure that everyone in the team has fair access to learning and development opportunities and support to improve their performance.

Managers will be asked to give examples of how they recognise the different needs of their staff and how they make sure all their staff have fair access to the support and learning and development opportunities they need.

Fair treatment and equality of access and opportunity are important in strengthening the psychological contract. Where employees can see that their manager ensures consistency of treatment and fairness they are more likely to respond by using the learning and development opportunities provided to improve their own and their team's performance. It is also consistent with the research from the '100 Best Companies to Work For' in that the work environment needs to support and challenge *all* staff to access the best in themselves. In addition in the modern day economy people are being encouraged to build a portfolio of skills and competencies to improve performance and also to make themselves more marketable.

Indicator 4: the capabilities managers need to lead, manage and develop people effectively are clearly defined and understood.
This indicator encourages organisations to be explicit in setting out the knowledge, skills and behaviours that are necessary for high performing management and to provide sufficient learning and development opportunities and support for managers to develop. By doing this it is acknowledging the key role that front line managers play in driving performance improvement. It also lets staff know what is reasonable for them to expect from their managers.

Do:

Indicators 5–8 Taking action to improve the performance of the organisation.

Indicator 5: managers are effective in leading, managing and developing people.
An IIP assessor will discuss with managers how they are effective in leading, managing and developing their staff. Clear examples will be required and these will be tested by separate discussions with staff. Staff will be asked to give examples of how they receive constructive feedback on their performance from their manager.

Whilst a formal appraisal system is not a requirement to achieve the IIP standard it is likely that within healthcare many managers will be working with an organisation wide appraisal system. Managers need support and training themselves in the 'soft skills' of conducting effective appraisal reviews and giving regular constructive feedback. Borill and West[8] showed that the extent and sophistication of appraisal was particularly strongly related to patient mortality.

This is also consistent with research on the psychological contract, staff want competent managers at work. It is also useful in highlighting the critical role of feedback from managers to their staff as outlined in the Healthcare Team Effectiveness Project.

Indicator 6: people's contribution to the organisation is recognised and valued. Maslow[4] highlighted the important contribution of recognition as a key means of improving satisfaction and commitment. Recognition of staff contribution has also been shown to be important in the '100 Best Companies to Work For' research and the Healthcare Team Effectiveness Project. It is a key skill for managers to celebrate success and recognise individual and team contribution. Staff need and want to know – not only how well they are doing – but that their efforts and achievements are being acknowledged and appreciated by their manager and the organisation. This can be done by managers taking the time to listen and respond positively to ideas and suggestions as well as finding the opportunities to say 'thank you' to their staff.

An IIP assessor will test out whether managers can give them examples of how they recognise and value the individual contribution of their staff and this will be cross-checked with what staff themselves say. Staff will also be asked to describe how they consider that they make a positive difference to the performance of the organisation.

Indicator 7: people are encouraged to take ownership and responsibility by being involved in decision making.
This is consistent with the demand from high performing organisations that staff are fully involved and make their contribution to decisions that formerly would have been seen as solely the responsibility of management. It demands a more participatory and collaborative management style from front line managers. Some managers need support and training themselves to adapt to this style.

Managers will be asked by an IIP assessor to give examples of how they promote a sense of 'ownership' and responsibility within their teams through involving staff appropriately in decision making. This also extends to trades unions and staff groups.

Staff will be asked to describe how they are encouraged to be involved in decision making that affects their own and their team's performance and how a sense of 'ownership' and responsibility is fostered by their manager.

Indicator 8: people learn and develop effectively.
This indicator encourages organisations to continually have mechanisms for evaluating the effectiveness of any learning and development activities. The key point is that staff put into practice what they have learnt in a way which will lead to performance improvement. Borrill and West[8] suggested that identifying and meeting training needs was one of the key HRM practices, which was associated with patient mortality.

Staff will be asked by an IIP assessor to describe how their learning and development needs have been met, what they have learnt and how they have put this into practice in their job. Similarly managers will be asked to give examples of how they make sure the learning and development needs of their staff are met and that their staff are putting their learning to good use and improving performance.

Review:

Indicators 9 and 10   Evaluating the impact on the performance of the organisation.

Indicator 9: investment in people improves the performance of the organisation. This is the indicator where many organisations struggle to produce the hard and soft evidence necessary to quantify the improvements at organisational and team levels to performance as a result of their investment in learning and development. It is usually easier for individual staff to quantify.

An IIP assessor will ask top managers to explain and quantify how learning and development has improved the performance of the organisation as well as how the evaluation of their investment in people is used to develop their strategy for improving performance.

Individual managers and staff will be asked to give examples of how learning and development has improved individual and team performance.

In healthcare, performance is measured through improved standards of patient care and outcomes. The work of Borrill and West[7,8] on the strong association between identifying and meeting training needs and providing feedback to improve performance and patient mortality points to a strong incentive for investment in people.

Indicator 10: improvements are continually made to the way people are managed and developed.

This indicator is encouraging an approach of continuous improvement. At every level it is encouraging a positive attitude to learning and development that leads to improved performance. It feeds into the IIP continuous circle of planning, doing and reviewing.

Top managers will be asked by the IIP assessor to give examples of how the evaluation of their investment in learning and development has led to improvements in their strategy for managing and developing their staff.

Managers will be asked by the IIP assessor to give examples of improvement they have made to how they manage and develop their staff. Asking staff to give examples of improvements that have been made to the way the whole organisation manages and develops staff tests this.

Conclusion

Modern HRM practice at a strategic level ensures that the people dimension is integral to organisational strategy. In healthcare, progressive HRM practices in particular appraisal, identifying and meeting training needs, feedback on performance and encouraging more team working, leads to improved performance and are strongly associated with patient mortality.

Where the psychological contract is positive, employee commitment and satisfaction will have a positive impact on business performance. Research demonstrates how important front line managers are in managing the psychological contract, delivering effective people management and bringing organisational policy and practice to life. Effective leadership of teams is an important aspect in motivating and managing people and an area for development in healthcare. Managers and leaders have an important role in creating an environment where staff will use their discretionary behaviour to give of their best and deliver improved patient care.

IIP is a leading benchmark standard for improving performance and ensuring that learning and development activities are planned, actioned and evaluated for staff at all levels of the organisation. It gives organisations an opportunity to compare their current polices and practices against a recognised benchmark and a structured way to improve the effectiveness of their training and developing activities. It moves away from the model of 'learning for learning's sake' to a model that emphasises performance improvement.

In an environment in which patients are becoming more knowledgeable and demanding and Government expectations are for year on year improvement there are ever greater expectations on managers. Their key role of managing staff and resources in ways that improve patient care, reduce patient mortality and retain motivated and committed staff is gaining a higher profile. There is a growing need for high quality management training in the softer skills of management to support managers in this key role.

Specific research in healthcare such as that carried out by the Healthcare Team Effectiveness Project is building a valuable evidence-base for managers to develop policy and practice in team working and other areas of HRM that will lead to real improvements and innovations in patient care. Further specific research projects are continuing with the NHS, for example 'Improving Health Through Human Resource Management, A Starting Point for Change'[11] focusing on the crucial role people management plays in the delivery of improvements and positive outcomes for patients in the NHS which is jointly commissioned by the DH, Association of Healthcare Human Resource Management and the Chartered Institute of Personnel and Development.

References

1 Guest D, Conway N. *Pressure at work and the psychological contract*. London: CIPD; 2002.
2 CIPD. *Factsheet: the psychological contract*. London: CIPD; 2007.
3 Leary-Joyce J. *Becoming an Employer of Choice*. London: CIPD; 2004.
4 Maslow A. A theory of human motivation. *Psychol Rev*. 1954; **50**: 370–96.
5 Katzenbach J, Smith D. *The Wisdom of Teams*. USA: Wiley; 1993.
6 Katzenbach J, Smith D. *The Discipline of Teams*. USA: Wiley; 2001.
7 Borrill C, West M, *et al. Team Working and Effectiveness in Health Care*. University of Aston, Birmingham. www.astonod.com.
8 Borrill C, West M, *et al. How Good is Your Team?* University of Aston, Birmingham. www.astonod.com.
9 West M, Borrill C, Dawson J, *et al.* The link between the management of employees and patient mortality in acute hospitals. *Int J Hum Res Manage*. 2002; **13**: 1299–310.
10 Investors in People. *Moving your organisation forward*. IIP Standard. London: HMSO; 2004.
11 CIPD. *Improving Health Through Human Resource Management A Starting Point for Change*. London: CIPD; 2006.

Chapter 6

Getting it right: the quality of care

Alan Gillies

What is quality?

Some of the simplest questions are the most difficult to answer. 'What is quality?' ranks with the most difficult of them. In domains such as engineering, quality is often linked to tangible physical properties. At least, it can be until you get people involved.

Consider three cars all associated with BMW, generally considered to be a 'quality' car producer.

These days, BMW own and produce Rolls-Royces. The very name Rolls-Royce is synonymous with quality in the mind of the general public. The name is used to describe other high quality products, for example, 'the Rolls-Royce of...'. Here, high quality is associated with a very high level of specification, a fast smooth ride, a high quality of finish on the paintwork, a great deal of hand craftsmanship, and a degree of perceived quality, otherwise known as 'snob-appeal'. The other key feature of the type of quality represented by the Rolls-Royce is that cost is no object. The aim is to produce the best possible car irrespective of price. Quality considerations related to economics are irrelevant. Criteria such as fuel economy, servicing intervals and costs and the price of insurance premiums are all irrelevant in this case. If you can afford the car, you can afford the rest. The Rolls-Royce represents quality in terms of excellence, unconstrained by cost considerations.

The BMW Series 3, on the other hand, is an example of a quality solution which epitomises a mass-produced product. Quality is still associated with the level of specification, quality of ride, quality of finish on the paintwork and so on, but expectations are lower and it is recognised that the product is designed to a price. Criteria connected with economics such as fuel economy, servicing intervals and costs and the price of insurance premiums are now some of the critical factors. Such cars are designed to provide the maximum quality at given cost.

The Mini brand is now also a BMW brand. The original Mini produced by British Leyland may not be regarded by some as a quality solution at all. It was unashamedly designed with cheapness in mind. All quality considerations were compromised by the cost factor. In absolute terms, the ride was poor, the comfort was poor, the speed performance was poor, but the car was cheap. Further, the car was cheap to maintain. Quality was compromised in areas such as comfort and ride and this may have been acceptable. The new Mini is more reliable but is more expensive to buy and to maintain.

However, if quality is compromised in the areas of reliability and maintainability, longer term costs are incurred and the overriding attraction of the car is lost. A cheap car with a limited specification is acceptable, but a cheap car that involves compromises that incur longer term expenditure is not a quality solution under any terms.

In almost every area, and patient care is certainly one of them, quality is intangible. As Kitchenham[1] said in a different context, quality in such cases is 'hard to define, impossible to measure, easy to recognise'.

Quality is most easily recognised in its absence and many public perceptions of healthcare are based upon measuring the absence of quality for example, waiting times, waiting list sizes, even illness itself are all measurements of the absence of quality.

Traditionally, quality has been seen as 'the degree of excellence'.[2] This is an attractive definition but is insufficient for our purposes. The nature of `excellence' must be considered in more detail to make the definition more effective. However, there is a more serious problem with this definition. Within a public health service context, it is necessary to consider the constraints upon excellence. Obviously, the primary constraint is budget, but others may exist, for example shortage of specialist skills in clinical specialities or nursing.

An alternative definition of quality is provided by the International Standards Organisation (ISO)[3] in 1986 as:

> The totality of features and characteristics of a product or service that bear on its ability to satisfy specified or implied needs.

The standard definition associates quality with the ability of the product or service to fulfil its function. It recognises that this is achieved through the features and characteristics of the product. Quality is associated both with having the required range of attributes and each achieving satisfactory performance within each attribute.

It is important to recognise some of the primary characteristics of quality:

- **quality is not absolute**. It means different things in different situations. In the case of cars, a Mini and Rolls-Royce both represent quality in different ways. Quality cannot be measured upon a quantifiable scale in the same way as physical properties such as temperature or length. Crucially in a service situation, people measure quality against their expectations. People's expectations of a Mini are not the same as they are of a Rolls-Royce. People's expectations of the modern Mini are quite different from their expectations of the old car
- **acceptable quality changes over time**. Expectations rise over time, no more so than in healthcare. Progress in clinical practice and improvements in care means that levels of performance deemed to be satisfactory are constantly being raised. This is an increase in both actual capability and in public expectation. People have expectations of the NHS in 2007 that they would not have dreamed of in 1997. This means they may get better service but still be more dissatisfied
- **quality is multidimensional**. It has many contributing factors. It is not easily summarised in a simple, quantitative way. Some aspects of quality can be measured objectively, for example, time spent waiting to see a doctor, some may not, for example quality of doctor's manner during a consultation. The most easily measured criteria are not necessarily the most important. People

are irrational beings and the acceptability of their treatment may depend upon criteria which are very hard to define

- **quality is subject to constraints**. Assessment of quality in most cases cannot be separated from cost. However, cost may be wider than simple financial cost: it refers to any critical resources such as people, tools and time. Some resources will be more constrained than others and where there is a high demand for a resource that is heavily constrained, the availability of that resource will become critical to overall quality. Healthcare is always rationed in any situation
- **quality is about acceptable compromises**. Where quality is constrained and compromises are required, some quality criteria may be sacrificed more acceptably than others; for example, comfort may be sacrificed before productivity. Those criteria that can least afford to be sacrificed may be regarded as critical attributes. They are often a small subset of the overall set of quality criteria
- **quality criteria are not independent**. The quality criteria are not independent, but interact with each other causing conflicts. For example, the greater the number of patients assigned to a clinic, the longer the waiting time during the clinic, but the shorter the waiting time to get an appointment. In this case, a conflict exists between the two desirable attributes.

Definitions from within healthcare

The problem of defining quality in healthcare terms is the complexity of the issue. Any domain where we are dealing with people rather than artefacts is infinitely more complex. This has caused many authors to say that looking at improving healthcare through a quality assurance model derived from manufacturing industry is inappropriate:

> Human well-being and the healthcare industry which deals with it are infinitely more complex than production lines.[4]

As far as it goes, this statement is fine, but quality assurance is now applied in many different organisational and service contexts which face many of the same issues as healthcare, for example education.

The difficulty is in not over simplifying the issues. This is particularly true when we seek to express the quality of healthcare in terms of simple quantitative measures.

For example, one traditional measure of healthcare is morbidity data. Many such measures tend to emphasise issues of quantity rather than quality. This tends to make health professionals uncomfortable who tend to evaluate themselves in terms of the quality of patients' lives rather than the quantity of it.

In practice, most writers in the clinical domain choose not to define quality at all, unless dealing with a very specific and tightly defined domain. For example, the definition of clinical audit provided by the Department of Health 1990[5] states:

> The systematic, critical analysis of the quality of medical care, including the procedures used for diagnosis and treatment, the use of resources and the resulting outcome and quality of life for the patient.

This definition contains the phrases 'quality of medical care' and 'quality of life' but nowhere defines what is meant by these terms. There is a broad consensus about general characteristics associated with these terms but at a detailed level, different clinicians and other interested parties, not least patients, are likely to disagree.

Therefore, rather than attempt a reductionist definition we shall consider different views of the quality of patient care in a specific context.

Quality is a multidimensional construct

We shall start by recognising that quality is a multidimensional construct. Therefore, it is perhaps inevitable that it has been classified according to a number of 'views' or perspectives. We shall represent this by a visual analogy, as shown in Figure 6.1.

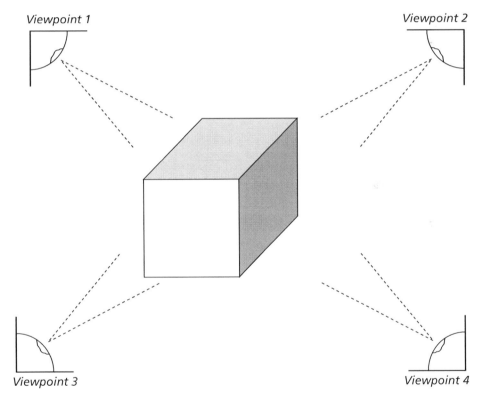

Figure 6.1 Visual analogy of quality as a multidimensional construct.

These views are often diverse and may conflict with each other. Each view comes from a particular context, and any single view tends to give us only a partial picture. The views identified tend to be stereotypical. For example, a distinction is commonly made within the Health Service context between clinicians or professionals and managers or administrators. The views are generally presented in adversarial pairs such as professionals versus administrators. Such comparisons are usually loaded by the terminology used.

Obviously, there are more than two people involved in any healthcare procedure. The long-term care of elderly patients is particularly problematic for a number of reasons:

- it involves an unusually large number of people in different roles dealing with the patient
- the patient may not be ill from an identifiable condition.

Let us consider an elderly person requiring physiotherapy. We shall consider each of the following roles and their view of quality:

- the client/patient
- the family
- the AHP
- the doctor
- the social worker
- the unit manager.

The client/patient: the client/patient's view of the quality of their experience will depend upon two factors: a successful outcome and a positive experience before, during and after treatment. The duality of this view is emphasised by the fact that most clients are not ill. Obviously at some points, these views are reinforcing. A simple and successful course of treatment which is minimally inconvenient and discomforting with a significant benefit in mobility and consequent improvements in the quality of life will encourage a positive view of the whole experience. However, some procedures which may be deemed clinically desirable to maximise the probability of a successful outcome may be highly uncomfortable and inconvenient for the patient.

Increasingly, the separation between these aspects is being questioned as it is recognised that clinical outcomes are influenced by a patient's general state of well-being. This increases the need to take account of what has been traditionally considered as non-clinical aspects of care.

The family: families generally have an immediate and longer-term interest in the process. As the client's family they have an interest in both the patient's health and happiness and will want what is best for their family member. However, they may incur significant inconvenience to support the client through the process. Decisions to exclude families from parts of the process on the grounds of clinical expediency can lead to dissatisfaction and resentment.

The AHP: the AHP is the primary provider of treatment. However, it will be part of a wider programme of care involving more healthcare professionals and hopefully an integrated multidisciplinary approach to care. There may be conflict with other professional groups who see the balance between intervention and outcomes differently. Also, all healthcare professionals are being influenced by a need to demonstrate that all eventualities were considered in the light of possible litigation in the event of problems.

The doctor: doctors are generally only involved significantly when there are clinical complications. This, coupled with the fact that the doctor carries responsibility for clinical problems will tend to emphasise a view of quality based upon clinical outcomes.

The social worker: the social worker may have responsibility for the wider care of the patient and wish to ensure that the programme of care fits alongside other services and support. This may be inconvenient in the short-term, but essential in the longer term to ensure that the client derives the maximum benefit from the care provided.

The unit manager: the manager of the unit – who may have a clinical or non clinical background – has the job of ensuring the quality of patient care delivered. Crucially, they have to weigh the needs of all patients rather than individuals. They have to weigh decisions against available resources and this leads to having to evaluate the quality of care against the quantity.

Within the general management context, Garvin[6] has suggested a model in terms of five different views of quality; see Figure 6.2:

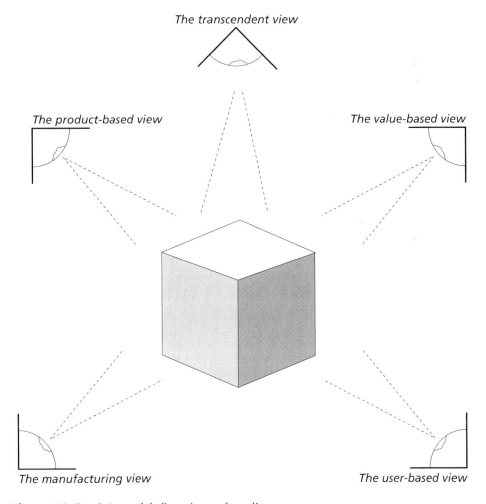

Figure 6.2 Garvin's model: five views of quality.

The meaning of Garvin's views are summarised in Table 6.1.

We shall now consider these views in more detail, within the context of healthcare.

Table 6.1 Summary of Garvin's views of quality.

View	Meaning
Transcendent	Absolute excellence
Product-based	Higher quality means higher cost
User-based	Fitness for purpose
Manufacturing	Conformance to specification
Value-based	Quality at a specific price

The transcendent view: this view relates quality to innate excellence. Another word for this might be 'elegance'. This is the classical definition of quality, in tune with the *Oxford English Dictionary*. It is impossible to quantify and is difficult to apply in a meaningful sense to healthcare. An attempt to build in a high degree of innate excellence to healthcare is likely to be constrained by resources. Seeking to build healthcare along these lines is inevitably expensive, and thus resource constraints will tend to emphasise the value-based view, described below, rather than the transcendent view.

The product-based view: this view is the economist's view: the higher the quality, the higher the cost. The basis for this view is that it costs money to provide a higher quality. This is a commonly held view about healthcare. Better care and quicker access to services are commonly linked to more doctors, nurses and hospital beds. However, in certain areas, better practice may also be cheaper. Examples of this may be found in screening programmes where health screening for example, for blood pressure, cervical cancer and child immunisation can actually save money in the long-term by keeping people healthy rather than treating people when they get ill.

Also, the growing practice of clinical audit is highlighting areas where practice can be improved without necessarily increasing costs.

This is the classic 'quality is free' argument proposed by the likes of Crosby[7] translated from manufacturing to healthcare. Crosby argues that by changing practice and reducing wastage, savings can be achieved in manufacturing which outweigh the costs of setting up the new procedures. However, unfortunately, this is by no means universal. Many improved practices will involve new technology requiring investment. Once wastage is removed, improvements in waiting lists can only be achieved by more resources.

Many of the screening programmes which are cost effective in the long-term are expensive in the short-term. For example, the growth in screening programmes in the UK has driven up computerisation rates amongst family doctors from around 25% to 90%. This represents a major investment whose cost must be set against the savings as illness is reduced.

Further, if screening programmes are justified on cost grounds alone, then programmes advantageous to health but less advantageous on cost grounds may be marginalised, for example breast cancer screening. From a health perspective, it is still better to prevent illness rather than treat it, but this case conforms to Garvin's product-based view, that is higher quality of care costs more.

The user-based view: this view was first championed by Juran[8] in the 1940s, is traditionally expressed as fitness for purpose. It is sometimes represented as patient satisfaction. This can however, be a simplification.

Fitness for purpose implies that the service provided meets the needs of patients. Thus, certain aspects of performance such as waiting times, access to services and patient satisfaction. However, overall fitness for purpose is compromised if waiting times are reduced by emphasising the treatment of conditions that are quick, easy and cheap at the expense of more seriously ill patients.

It is also compromised if waiting times are reduced at the expense of reducing the effectiveness of treatment provided leading to an increase in re-admissions. Many measures currently applied to the UK NHS which purport to measure NHS fitness for purpose, for example waiting times, waiting list sizes, number of patients treated, actually measure the quantity of healthcare provided rather than the quality.

The manufacturing view: the manufacturer's view measures quality in terms of conformance to requirements. A simple example might be the dimensions of a component. The specification will state both the required dimension and the tolerance that will be acceptable.

The manufacturing view emerges in healthcare in a number of ways. One way is the introduction of protocols and standards for specific clinical procedures. These may be regarded as a specification for a clinical procedure. In the UK, one of the stated outcomes of the clinical audit process is the introduction of standards to disseminate 'best practice'.

However, the setting of such standards is by no mean universal; a report on audit practice in the Oxfordshire Health Authority revealed that only 46% of audits were claimed to result in the setting of standards. Evaluation of 75 published audits indicated a 41% uptake. As published audits, these may be expected to show a higher uptake than the whole, suggesting that the real figure may be lower.

In practice, it is rarely possible to provide guidelines which embody 'best practice'. Guidelines will prevent bad practice and can lead to uniform improvements where existing practice is flawed. However, best practice generally requires skills and judgement which are not easily enshrined in deterministic procedures. Thus the result of guidelines can be problem avoidance rather than promotion of excellence.

Best practice requires the exercising of judgement, rather than following a deterministic procedure. The biggest threat to this lies in the increasing threat of malpractice suits. This encourages practitioners to view quality in terms of meeting a specification. If the specification is met, the doctor has fulfilled his obligation, even if the patients' aspirations are not met.

The value-based view: in a business context, this is the ability to provide what the customer requires at a price that they can afford. In a public health service, the customer is ultimately the taxpaying public represented by the Government. A value-based view of quality assesses the cost effectiveness of a service or treatment.

The value-based view is the antithesis of the transcendent view, because it links quality to cost. Within the management of quality in the NHS context, this is often the crucial view. It is also what tends to give NHS management a bad name in the eyes of the public, as it recognises that quality is ultimately resource-limited. Although there are cases where better healthcare costs less not more as described above, in general this is not the case.

Garvin's model is not necessarily appropriate for healthcare. For example, the manufacturing view which is dominant in many areas of traditional quality management is of limited use. The author therefore proposes an alternative view-based model of quality for healthcare; see Figure 6.3.

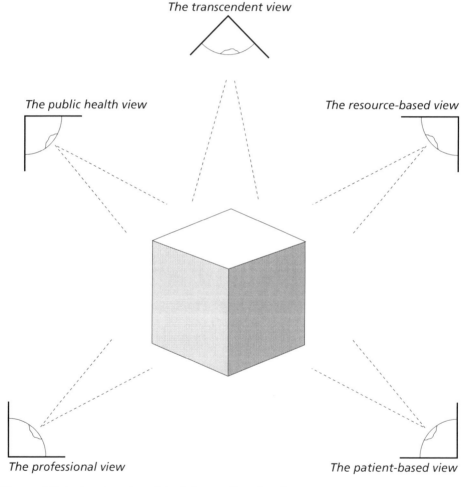

Figure 6.3 A view-based model of the quality of patient care.

The transcendent view: this view is the same as Garvin's. It is included because it is such a deeply ingrained view of quality. It is little help in analysing the problem of improving the quality of patient care. However, it is important to recognise its crucial place in many people's understanding of the nature of quality.

The public health view: this view is based upon the view that the quality of patient care is demonstrated by the health of the nation. It is the view at the heart of the UK Government's strategy document 'Health of the Nation' which sets targets for key areas of health to be achieved by the end of the decade.

A key element of this view is that quality of care is reflected in maintaining and restoring health rather than through treating illness. This view may be seen as a strategic view of the quality of patient care.

The resource-based view: the resource-based view says that the quality of patient care is the maximum care that can be obtained for the resources allocated by the country to public healthcare. Thus it is concerned with the effectiveness of patient care, reduction of waste and promotion of best practice measured in terms of value for money. This may be thought of as the management view, at both an operational and strategic level.

The professional view: this view emphasises clinical outcomes and clinical expertise. It sets a successful clinical outcome as the primary measure of success. Traditionally, it has emphasised the central role of the doctor. It is increasingly coming to promote a team-based approach. However, some doctors may use a narrow form of this view to resist change in this direction. It is a view associated with doctors and other clinical professionals.

The patient-based view: the patient-based view says that the patients' overall well-being and satisfaction is crucial. It tends to an individualistic view rather than a collective vision, as the needs of each patient may be different and conflict under the resource-based view with the needs of other patients. It may in certain cases conflict with the professional view as well. However, many professionals placing their patients' needs as their prime objective, will subscribe to this view, although expressing in a different way from the patients they seek to serve.

These views are necessarily stereotypical, as any model must represent a subset of reality. They are intended to be less stereotypical than a reductionist definition and more appropriate to healthcare than Garvin's general model.

Conflicts and constraints

There is an extra degree of complexity inherent in this model which arises from the relationships which exist between each view of quality. It is suggested that each of the views except the transcendent view is in dynamic equilibrium with the others. The equilibrium is dynamic because many improvements as perceived from one point of view may degrade quality when perceived from another view. Each of the other four contributes to the transcendent view.

The dynamic equilibrium may be thought of in terms of a variety of conflicts between different views; see Figure 6.4.

The most commonly considered conflict is between cost and quality, or in terms of our views between the resource-based view and the public health view. Any improvements which can impact positively on more than one view without negatively impacting elsewhere are particularly attractive. Some of the screening programmes mentioned earlier are in this category.

However, there are other conflicts at work between the different views. There is a significant and growing conflict between patient and professional-based

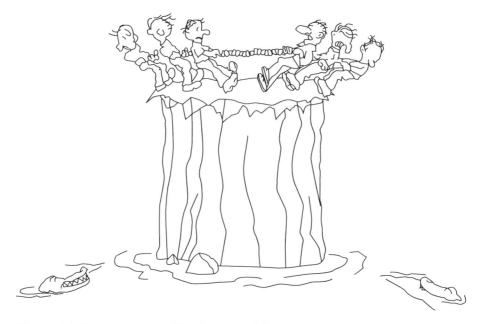

Figure 6.4 There may be conflicts between different views.

views. A better informed public arising from a more patient-centred approach argues more strongly for their rights and attacks the traditionally unquestioned expertise of the professionals.

Part of this is a growing awareness of the right of patients to make charges of negligence in cases where things go wrong. This has a number of consequences, but one is that doctors may take courses of action in order to protect themselves against malpractice suits rather than for patient-centred reasons. This will then tend to reduce the quality in terms of the patient-based approach. This has been seen much more in the US, where litigation is much more common than in the UK.

An example may be seen in the behaviour of American obstetricians, who in the face of increasing incidence of malpractice suits over birth canal deliveries opted for an increased number of caesarean section deliveries. In spite of the increased risk to patients, this was less likely to lead to a law suit. At its peak, this trend led to approximately 50% of births being delivered in this way.

However, this was followed by a series of law suits which alleged unnecessary caesarean operations, which in turn reduced the number of operations. This slightly bizarre example illustrates the dynamic equilibrium which exists between different views of quality.

In an ideal world, all views would be satisfied, leading to the transcendent view of quality. However, in the real world, all of the others exist in different degrees of tension with each other. This is what makes a discussion of the quality of patient care so difficult and makes a multidimensional treatment essential.

Clinical audit

Clinical audit is a process by which we can measure our clinical practice against a 'gold standard'.

Clinical audit was introduced in 1989 in the Department of Health White Paper *Working for Patients*.[9] Since then the scope has been extended to nursing (1990) and subsequently to all healthcare professions. Audit has been recognised as an activity involving all healthcare workers and hence the term has changed from medical audit to clinical audit to recognise this.

The process of clinical audit is defined in the audit cycle (Figure 6.5) which shows a remarkable similarity to classical process improvement techniques pioneered by Deming and Shewhart (see Chapter 4 of Gillies[10]).

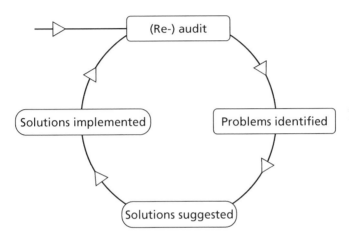

Figure 6.5 The clinical audit cycle.

Audit is not new. Aside from its links to process improvement, it may trace its roots back through the attempts of clinicians to improve their professional activities, for example:

- 1858: improved management of basic care: Florence Nightingale
- 1916: definition of standards and the need for confidentiality by Bowman and the US College of Surgeons
- 1952: voluntary collection of standard data on maternal mortality: UK Ministry of Health.

More information on this is provided in Chapter 2 of Gillies.[10]

Clinical audits have a number of characteristics which most will share. They are locally organised and controlled. They are generally small scale and have the stated aim of improving patient care. The latter is normally a condition of funding. Clinical audit is a 'bottom up' approach to quality management.

Crucially, audit should result in changes in practice to effect change. They should be carried out in a systematic manner. They should be an ongoing process, or at the very least contain a commitment to re-audit to investigate the effect of changes.

The Department of Health definition from the 1989 White Paper[9] sets out the desirable characteristics of the audit process. Audit should be:

- systematic

- analytical
- concerned with the quality of care.

This statement also outlines the scope of audit activity. It should cover:

- procedures for diagnosis and treatment
- the use of resources
- the resulting outcomes
- the impact upon the quality of life of the patient.

Audits are carried out by many different people from many different backgrounds. It is questionable whether the overall approach to clinical audit is indeed systematic and analytical. Individual audits show a wide variation in the techniques used and the scope considered.

The purpose of clinical audit is to assist in the management of patient care and to identify problems and to facilitate improvement. Clinical audit differs from other forms of audit in a number of key ways:

- it is perceived to be about a process of improvement rather than a snapshot of current performance
- it is carried out at different levels within the organisation, often initiated by local practitioners at their own level
- it is not an overall process of quality assurance imposed from outside in the way that, for example, inspection of education is carried out.

This has a number of clear advantages in terms of user involvement and ownership. It greatly increases the enthusiasm of the practitioners for the process who perceive it as helpful in general rather than authoritarian.

The ideal form of clinical audit proposed by the White Paper is in fact far from ideal as a quality management procedure. Many of the limitations, however, may still reflect the fact that clinical audit is an optimal solution to a trade-off between two conflicting goals.

For example, in order to facilitate change, it is essential to establish local ownership and direction of projects. However, this reduces the effectiveness of audit as a tool for management. Many SHAs have no central records of the number and nature of audits carried out. Local control implies a lack of central control. This changes the role of audit to a tool which feeds into operational management rather than strategic management.

There is an inherent trade-off between local control and strategic effectiveness.

Another conflict may be seen as the focus of an audit. It has been stated that audits should be focused, not open ended as in research. However, it is also suggested that audit should deal in underlying causes, not symptoms if real improvements are to be achieved. This may not be possible if the approach adopted is too focused.

The use of computers has already highlighted the danger of too much focus on data collection and analysis at the expense of implemented change. At the same time, poor data will fail to deliver real improvement in practice.

Finally, there is the ultimate tension of best use of resources. If a clinician is overloaded, how far is it justified in increasing the problem by reducing his or her time to see patients by involving them in an audit to try to identify root causes of the problem?

Clinical governance

Since 1 April 1999, clinical governance has been a required part of the activity of NHS organisations such as hospital Trust primary care groups and health authorities. The publicity given to scandals such as those in Bristol and Kent has ensured a high priority for this activity (see the first book in this series *Managing and Leading in the Allied Health Professions*, Chapters 8 and 9).

In 1997, following the election of a new Government, as part of the new wave of NHS reforms clinical governance was introduced as a systematic process of quality assurance.[11] Whilst this was being discussed, a major scandal broke in Bristol, which has forced the external scrutiny of professional practice to be introduced.[12,13]

Clinical governance is much more ambitious in scope than clinical audit. It emphasises quality assurance much more than quality improvement. It is intended to cover all aspects of the NHS. NHS documents describe clinical governance as a quality assurance process where quality assurance is defined as: the use of a monitoring system to measure performance against quality standards.[14]

Thus, the view of quality being emphasised is the manufacturing view, with practice measured against a specified target.

Whilst clinical governance was still being developed, the environment in which it was to operate was radically changed by a major scandal in paediatric cardiac surgery at Bristol Royal Infirmary. The longest inquiry ever held by the GMC found that the deaths of 29 babies were due to the gross negligence of the doctors involved resulting in two doctors being struck off the medical register and a third being suspended.

The case generated a huge public outcry and undoubtedly shifted the UK healthcare quality assurance agenda. Smith[13] argued that:

> The Bristol case, in which judgement was passed last week will probably prove much more important to the future of healthcare in Britain than the reforms suggested in the White Papers. Reorganisations of the NHS come round with monotonous regularity, but changes on the wards and in surgeries are slow and often unrelated to the passing political rhetoric. In contrast, the Bristol case is a once in a lifetime drama that has held the attention of doctors and patients in a way that a White Paper can never hope to match.

There is evidence of other major catastrophes such as major fires shifting public policy by a major step change. Smith predicted the major impact upon professional practice that has seen significant reductions in clinical professional autonomy and increases in regulation of professional practice.

However, if we focus on its impact upon the implementation on clinical governance then it has a number of specific consequences, which may be counter-productive.

- it focuses on a view of quality which is designed to prevent catastrophic failure rather than provide general improvement
- it has made it acceptable to scrutinise professional practice
- it emphasises a view that clinical governance is about weeding out 'bad practitioners'

- it encourages defensive practice and therefore discourages innovation and improvement
- it may discourage clinicians from practising in high risk areas and with high risk patients: all of the child patients in the Bristol case were in this category.

In 2006, Sir Ian Kennedy who chaired the inquiry into Bristol reflected on progress since the inquiry:

> As the acting Chief Executive of the NHS, Sir Ian Carruthers, made clear in his first Report in June, 2006, there has been a range of improvements in the service offered to patients by the NHS. As the leader in the *Guardian* put it the next day, Sir Ian set out 'dramatic improvements on a succession of health fronts: hospital inpatient waiting times down to record low levels; outpatient access radically improved; accident and emergency care targets (once regarded as impossible) now being met; and the management of chronic care transformed by 1000 community matrons …

Then there were the statistics on what this meant for patients. Steep drops in mortality numbers from the two biggest killers – coronary disease and cancer – with the NHS on target to deliver a 40% reduction in cardiovascular deaths in people under-75 by 2010. There were other good news stories on preventive health, the reduction of suicides and new moves to reduce health inequalities. That is the picture from the inside and reflects real progress.

> There was some justification, therefore, for the Secretary of State to say in May 2006 that the NHS had had its best year yet, as regards the care and treatment of patients (which, after all, is what it is all about). The obsession of particular sections of society with a limited (although not unimportant) set of examples of poor financial management, or with what is called (without analysis) privatisation, should not be allowed to obscure the successes achieved. These are, of course, the consequence, in part, of Government's policies. They are also, in part, the consequence of those going to work every day to make things happen, sometimes because of and sometimes in spite of Government's policies. So, the Secretary of State had a point: she should, however, and no doubt, would have gone on to agree that there still remains so much more to do.[15]

Under current clinical governance arrangements, the Healthcare Commission is responsible for the quality of care within the NHS. Each year, they produce an annual report. The 2006 report, that Sir Ian cites, argues that quality is getting better and points to areas that still need improvement:

> The quality of care is improving too. Fewer people are dying from cancer and heart disease, thanks in part to better quality care. More women are screened and treated for breast cancer earlier, when they have a better chance of surviving the disease. Wider use of statins (drugs used to lower cholesterol) is helping to reduce the risk of heart disease. In England and Wales, more patients with mental health problems are getting better support so that they can live in the community. We have also found some improvements in services to help people to quit smoking, particularly in disadvantaged areas.[16]

In 2005, there were almost 14 million out-patient appointments and 18 million attendances for emergency care. The majority of patients experience safe healthcare and there is evidence of improvements in safety. For example, 75% of staff say that their Trust encourages them to report incidents and fewer staff are reporting seeing error or near misses (40% in 2005, down from 47% in 2003).

> However, our work shows that some healthcare organisations, in both the public and private sector, need a more consistent emphasis on safety on behalf of patients. One in ten healthcare organisations could not assure us that they fully met all the standards relating to safety – although this doesn't mean that they are unsafe. Each year we receive almost 8,000 complaints which have not been resolved by NHS Trusts. Of these, one-fifth are safety related. There are also widely different estimates of the number of avoidable deaths of patients, and the number of serious injuries, that occur each year. Any unnecessary harm is too much. We are concerned that, as a country, we do not have reliable information. This type of information is crucial to avoiding adverse incidents and their effects in the future. All developed countries face similar challenges.[16]

Providing the best possible care

In terms of the quality of care provided by individual professionals we may consider two aspects, derived from the ethical codes which underpin all clinical practice, do the most good and do no harm.

In order to do the most good, professionals have an obligation to keep their practice up to date. The HPC require the registrants to maintain quality by adhering to personal standards in the areas of character, health, proficiency, conduct, performance and ethics, and to ensure that their practice continues to meet these standards through continuing professional development.[17]

Box 6.1 HPC standards of proficiency.

The registrants are required to:
1 demonstrate professional autonomy and accountability by:
  - being able to practice within the legal and ethical boundaries of their profession
  - being able to practice in a non-discriminatory manner
  - being able to maintain confidentiality and obtain informed consent
  - being able to exercise a professional duty of care
  - knowing the limits of their practice and when to seek advice
  - recognising the need for effective self-management of workload and be able to practice accordingly
  - understanding the obligation to maintain fitness to practice
  - understanding the need for career-long self-directed learning.
2 establish and maintain professional relationships by:
  - knowing the professional and personal scope of their practice and be able to make referrals

- being able to work, where appropriate, in partnership with other professionals, supporting staff, patients, clients and users, and their relatives and carers
- being able to contribute effectively to work undertaken as part of a multi-disciplinary team
- being able to demonstrate effective and appropriate skills in communicating information
- giving advice, instruction and professional opinion to colleagues, patients, clients, users, their relatives and carers
- understanding the need for effective communication throughout the care of the patient, client or user.

3 identify and assess health and social care needs by:
- being able to gather appropriate information
- being able to use appropriate assessment techniques
- being able to undertake or arrange clinical investigations as appropriate
- being able to analyse and evaluate the information collected.

4 formulate and deliver plans and strategies for meeting health and social care needs by:
- being able to use research, reasoning and problem solving skills
- being able to draw on appropriate knowledge and skills in order to make professional judgements
- being able to formulate specific and appropriate management plans including the setting of time scales
- being able to conduct appropriate diagnostic or monitoring procedures, treatment, therapy or other actions safely and skilfully
- being able to maintain records appropriately.

5 critically evaluate the impact of, or response to, the registrant's actions by:
- being able to monitor and review the ongoing effectiveness of planned activity and modify it accordingly
- being able to audit, reflect on and review practice
- the skills required for the application of practice.

6 maintain the knowledge, skills and understanding required for their role by:
- knowing the key concepts of the biological, physical, social, psychological and clinical sciences which are relevant to their profession-specific practice
- knowing how professional principles are expressed and translated into action through a number of different approaches to practice, and how to select or modify approaches to meet the needs of an individual
- understanding the need to establish and maintain a safe practice environment.

Starting in 2006, the Council has implemented a process of auditing professional development of registered professionals to ensure compliance. See Table 6.2. It's coming your way soon!

Table 6.2 Auditing cycle for AHPs.

July 2008	Chiropodists and podiatrists
October 2008	Operating department practitioners
August 2009	Orthoptists
August 2009	Paramedics
September 2009	Clinical scientists
September 2009	Prosthetists and orthotists
September 2009	Speech and language therapists
October 2009	Occupational therapists
November 2009	Biomedical scientists
February 2010	Radiographers
April 2010	Physiotherapists
May 2010	Arts therapists
May 2010	Dietitians

Editors' note

For further reading on legal issues arising in the management, leadership and development of AHP, professional regulation and clinical governance see the first book in this series *Managing and Leading in the Allied Health Professions.*[18]

Preventing harm

A major part of quality healthcare is ensuring that as professionals we do not do harm to patients or clients. In spite of this, there are a very high number of adverse events in the NHS, and many of them lead to harm to patients.

The majority of incidents reported to the National Reporting and Learning System (NRLS) (69%) involved no harm to patients, and 25% involved only minor or minimal harm. A further 5% involved moderate – but no permanent – harm, 0.9% involved severe permanent harm and 0.4% (2159 cases in total) involved the death of a patient.

> The survey by the National Audit Office found a similar number of deaths (2181). However, these figures only reflect incidents that were identified and reported. There are many other cases in which an aspect of care might have contributed to or hastened the death of a patient – up to 40 000 each year, according to one study. In some of these cases, the people who died had been very seriously ill and the most effective course of action may not have been clear.[16]

The 2005 NHS Staff survey of 33 000 AHPs found significant evidence of harm to patients through adverse events. The survey reported the following findings for AHPs within the NHS (Box 6.2).

Box 6.2 NHS staff survey 2005 – AHP findings.

- 30% reported seeing errors, near misses or incidents that could hurt patients/service users in the last month.
- 22% reported seeing errors, near misses or incidents that could hurt staff.
- 14% of those who had seen an error, near miss or incident, failed to report it.
- 40% agreed or strongly agreed that their Trust treats fairly staff who are involved in an error, near miss or incident.
- 77% agreed or strongly agreed that their Trust encourages staff who are involved in an error, near miss or incident to report it.
- 51% agreed or strongly agreed that their Trust treats reports of errors, near misses or incidents confidentially.
- 5% agreed or strongly agreed that their Trust blames or punishes people who make errors, near misses or incidents.
- 45% agreed or strongly agreed that when errors, near misses or incidents are reported their Trust takes action to ensure that they do not happen again.
- 25% agreed or strongly agreed that their Trust informed them about errors, near misses and incidents that happen in their Trust.
- 28% agreed or strongly agreed that their Trust provides feedback about changes made in response to reported errors, near misses and incidents.

Who is responsible for quality?

So who is responsible for the quality of care? No amount of regulation from the Healthcare Commission or the HPC can detract from the fact that ultimately the quality of care is controlled by those who deliver it.

Every healthcare practitioner has responsibility to do the best they can, to ensure that their practice meets, or preferably exceeds, the standards described by their Regulator and Professional Body. It is important to continually learn from successes and mistakes and to provide the best possible quality of care.

How do we know if what we do is good enough? Try the mother test.

If your mother is the patient or client receiving care or treatment, would you think it is good enough? If so, it's probably good enough. If not, why is it good enough for someone else's mother?

References

1 Kitchenham B. Software quality assurance, *Microprocessor & Microcomputers*.1989; **13**(6): 373–81.
2 *Oxford English Dictionary*. 2nd ed. Oxford: Oxford University Press; 1989.
3 International Standards Organisation. ISO8042: Quality Vocabulary, Geneva: ISO; 1986.
4 Crombie I, Davies H, Abraham S, *et al. The Audit Handbook: improving healthcare through clinical audit.* Chichester: John Wiley; 1993.
5 Department of Health. Framework for information systems: overview, working for patients. Working Paper 11. London: HMSO; 1990.

6 Garvin D. What does product quality mean? *Sloan Management Review*.1984; **1**: 25-41.

7 Crosby PB. *Quality is Free*. 2nd ed. London: McGraw-Hill; 1986.

8 Juran JM. *Quality Control Handbook*. 3rd edn. London: McGraw-Hill; 1979.

9 Department of Health. Working for Patients. London: HMSO; 1989.

10 Gillies AC. *Improving the Quality of Patient Care*. Chichester: Wiley; 1997.

11 Department of Health. The New NHS White Paper. London: HMSO; 1997.

12 Dyer C. British doctors found guilty of serious professional misconduct. *BMJ*. 1998; **316**: 1924.

13 Smith R. All changed, changed utterly. *BMJ*. 1989; **316**: 1917–18.

14 NHSE North Thames. Clinical Governance, Discussion Paper (Revision 6). London: Department of Health; 1998.

15 Kennedy I. Learning from Bristol: are we? London: Health Care Commission; 2006.

16 Health Care Commission. State of Health Care. London: Commission for Healthcare Audit and Inspection; 2006.

17 Health Professions Council. Physiotherapy, Standards of proficiency. London: HPC; 2005.

18 Jones R, Jenkins F. *Managing and Leading in the Allied Health Professions*. Oxford: Radcliffe Press; 2006.

Chapter 7

User involvement in services for disabled people

Sally French and John Swain

The concept of user involvement is now well established within managerial practice and enshrined in legislation. It is no longer the case that managers can or should make decisions on behalf of those they serve.

Robson *et al*[1] define user involvement as:

> ... the participation of users of services in decisions that affect their lives.

Croft and Beresford[2] believe that:

> Speaking and acting for yourself and being part of mainstream society, lies at the heart of social care service user involvement.

Though the concept of user involvement is well established, it remains fraught with controversy and problematic issues. Perhaps the most fundamental questions, reverberating through all levels of service provision, address the 'who' and 'why' of user involvement. In simple terms, is it motivated, generated and managed by service users? Or is it motivated, generated and managed by service managers? An institution, organisation or service can, in the present cultural climate, be given enhanced credibility through its public face of user involvement.

In this chapter user involvement in the health and social services will be discussed focusing on disabled people. It will commence with a brief historical overview of user involvement in health and social care services. Some methods of user involvement will then be described and the chapter will conclude with an examination of the various barriers which impede user involvement by disabled people and how these may be removed or minimised. The discussion throughout will explore the implications for the management of health and social care services.

The development of user involvement

The development of user involvement in services for disabled people arose in Britain in two main ways. Following the election of Margaret Thatcher as Conservative Prime Minister in 1979, there was a shift towards a market ideology in health and social care (see the first book in this series *Managing and Leading in the Allied Health Profession* Chapter 2). A quasi-market was introduced into health and social services to allow some degree of choice for patients and clients who were now regarded as consumers. The idea was that services would be 'needs-led' rather than 'service-led' and that disabled people and other service users would be assessed for individual 'packages of care' within a 'mixed economy of welfare' including private, voluntary and statutory services.[3,4]

These changes were backed by legislation and various policy documents from the Department of Health, including the Children Act of 1989[5] and the NHS and Community Care Act of 1990.[6] User consultation and collaboration in service planning and delivery was made mandatory in these Acts. Managers were, for example, required to consult with consumers regarding community care plans. This reflected the consumerist ideology of the political right and was viewed as a way of cutting costs, providing more flexible services and reducing state involvement as well as the power of professionals.[7] In 1997 these policies were, in essence, continued in New Labour's modernisation agenda for health and social care.[8,9] Barriers to the inherent change in power relations between service providers, managers and service users were widely identified. People who are powerless and marginalised within society may not be able readily to express themselves, to make complaints or to effect change. O'Sullivan[10] states that:

> A principle of sound decision-making practice is for clients to have the highest feasible level of involvement, but they may not always feel sufficiently empowered to make decisions ... Stakeholders need to consult with each other to share information but the presence of clients at these meetings is not sufficient in itself to ensure their involvement. Active steps may be required to prevent them being excluded from meaningful participation.

One clear strategy in the face of barriers to service user involvement has been the alignment of people with power to those who are powerless in order to help them express their needs and concerns. It follows from this that independent advocacy is an essential service when considering user involvement including the provision and accessibility of information. The need for advocacy is also enshrined within government policy. For example in the White Paper on mental health, 'Reforming the Mental Health Act'[11] it is stated:

> Under new legislation providers of health and social care services will be required to ensure that patients who are subject to care and treatment under compulsory powers have access to independent specialist advocacy services ... health authorities will ensure suitable independent advocacy is made available ... The role of specialist advocates will be to provide information and, if appropriate, help the patient represent his or her views in discussions with the clinical team about his or her care or treatment under formal powers.

Croft and Beresford[7] make the point that 'empowerment' has become a key concept in social care which is central to political, social policy, educational and managerial discourses.

As a result of these changes in ideology, policy and legislation, the 1990s saw a considerable growth in user involvement initiatives particularly in the social services where thousands of disabled people now participate in a range of activities.[12] Few initiatives, however, have been thoroughly evaluated and many have proved ineffective.[13,9] Robson *et al*[1] and Carr[9] note the lack of research, monitoring and evaluation with regard to the impact and outcome of user participation. Agencies tend to focus on the benefits of participation itself rather than on the outcomes achieved, sometimes even viewing participation as a form of 'therapy' to improve the skills, competence and self-esteem of disabled people.[14] Carr[9] states:

> There is a general lack of research and evaluation on the impact and outcomes of service user participation. Little seems to be formally recorded at local, regional or national levels and the influence of user participation on transforming services has not been the subject of any major UK research studies.

A further development that took place during the 1970s and 1980s was the emergence of well organised and strengthening user movements including the Disabled People's Movement. The agenda of this goes far beyond the issue of services (however important they may be) to full democratic citizenship and the dismantling of a disabling environment in terms of physical and social barriers.[15,16] Other social movements, such as Survivors Speak Out, Gay Pride, and the Self Advocacy Movement have similar agendas. Talking of the Disabled People's Movement Drake[17] states that:

> ... it is important to give due weight to the contribution that the disability movement has made in changing the thinking of governments, bringing injustice to light and forcing a radical alteration of the policy agenda.

Carr[9] also stresses the importance of collectivism in user involvement for disabled people and the ideas and philosophy of the social model of disability which underpin it.

Standing back from these two ways that service user involvement has developed, there are clear contradictions and controversies that reverberate through issues of management. Beresford and Croft[7] note the tension between the ideologies of the government and those of the Disabled People's Movement. They state:

> These two approaches to participation, the consumerist and democratic approaches, do not sit comfortably. One is managerial and instrumental in purpose, without any commitment to the redistribution of power or control, the other liberational with a commitment to empowerment.

Brown[18] emphasises the depth of this conflict:

> Service users have not only focused on the way they want services delivered but also challenged the relevance and appropriateness of the knowledge base upon which professionals traditionally draw. User movements have increasingly been involved in generating theory about their position in the world – theory which rests on the analysis and lived experience of people who use health and social care services.

In addressing the inherent tensions, Beresford *et al*[13] and Priestley[19] emphasise that user involvement is merely a vehicle for effective change in terms of the services delivered and the behaviour of those who deliver them. Similarly Carmichael[12] stresses that:

> User involvement is a means to an end and not an end in itself.

In terms of legislation it can be argued that a framework for change is being established. The Disability Discrimination Act,[20] the Human Rights Act[21] and the Disability Rights Bill[22] will, perhaps, go some way in assisting disabled people in their struggle for full participative citizenship. Article ten of the European Convention of Human Rights[23] established the right to self-expression and article six established the right to a fair hearing. The power of legislation to bring about change is, however, frequently exaggerated as is apparent in the continuing discrimination against ethnic minorities and women despite the passing of anti-discrimination Acts some thirty years ago.

Methods of user involvement

Methods of involving users of services can take many forms. Brown[18] lists the following methods:

- residents' committees
- user panels
- customer surveys
- suggestion boxes
- involvement in management committees
- involvement in forums and working parties
- focus groups
- public meetings.

Goss and Miller[24] depict user involvement as a ladder with the top rung giving total control to users and the bottom rung giving no control at all.

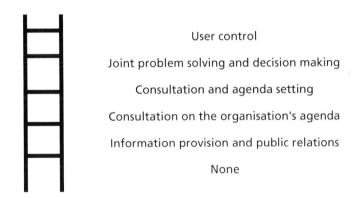

User control

Joint problem solving and decision making

Consultation and agenda setting

Consultation on the organisation's agenda

Information provision and public relations

None

Figure 7.1 Ladder of user involvement – adapted from Goss and Miller.[24]

Bewley and Glendinning[25] warn against relying heavily on any one method or model as none are perfect and a variety are needed to reach all disabled people. They note a heavy reliance on formal meetings in user involvement and point out that in order to reach black disabled people, people living in rural areas and other marginalised groups, such as travellers, people with mental health problems and people with learning difficulties, a community development approach, working with local networks, needs to be adopted on a sustained basis. Carr[9], in her review of the literature, found that little attention was paid to the diversity of users even though those from ethnic minorities were often in most need of services. She also found that the belief that disabled people from ethnic minorities 'look after their own' – and therefore do not need services – is still prevalent. The inequalities in health and social services that people from ethnic minority groups experience have been well documented.[26,27]

Service user involvement, as generated within the development of the Disabled People's Movement and broader context of user movements, needs to be understood within a wide range of strategies for social change and the management of changing power relations between service providers/managers and service users. Such strategies include direct action, lobbying and the provision of disability equality training, controlled and delivered by disabled people. Research has a role to play, perhaps particularly with the emphasis placed on evidence-based practice. Service user involvement, however, remains of paramount importance.

Regarding research, it is essential that disabled people are centrally involved, not just to give their responses to questions, but to decide on the research agenda, the methodology and how the research will be used. Swain and French [28] state:

> Many disabled people are of the opinion that medically orientated research has not fundamentally altered their position within society ... the way in which disability has been researched has become a major issue for disabled people and their organisations in recent times.

Service user organisations have contributed to the growing body of research into health and social care service provision. These are user-led research initiatives. One example is a research project examining people's experience of mental health services, resulting in the report 'Strategies for Living'.[29]

Evans and Fisher[30] suggest that the management team's positive contribution to developing service user involvement processes is a key factor in its success. Writing of the Wiltshire and Swindon Service Users Network, they found that service users were involved in a number of ways including:

- initiating the idea of evaluation
- participating with managers in a working group
- suggesting a survey of service users
- helping devise an accessible questionnaire
- contributing to discussions about dissemination of service users' views
- participating in local quality groups
- training
- service monitoring.

Barriers to user participation

Many practical, organisational and cultural barriers need to be addressed if the involvement of disabled people in the management, planning and delivery of health and social care services is to become a reality. A central issue is the unequal power relationship between service users and professionals and managers.[31] Priestley states that:

> It is impossible to discuss user participation without reference to power. If providers are committed to increasing user power then they must contemplate a corresponding reduction of their own power.

The power imbalance between disabled people on the one hand and professionals and managers on the other, extends to the meaning of important concepts that affect disabled people's lives. Disabled people and professionals tend, for example, to have a very different idea of the meaning of 'care' and 'independence' with the view of professionals and managers predominating and being translated into policy and practice.[9,32,33] Disabled people prefer the notion of 'support' rather than 'care' where they are in control of the help provided. Similarly, they view 'independence', not as being able to do everything for themselves, but being in control of their lives. Beresford et al[34] believe that users of services need to be involved in defining the meaning of 'quality' as their definition is fundamentally different from that of service managers and agencies. Views about quality in services are based upon cultural and professional assumptions which are underpinned by paternalism rather than on the perspectives of those who use the services which are based on rights.[13]

A further way in which inequality of power is apparent in health and social care services is in the setting of agendas for the planning of those services. These are usually set by professionals and managers rather than disabled people themselves.[9] Therapists may, for example, decide how to organise their work in the community without consulting with those they will serve. Furthermore the involvement of disabled people is usually dependent upon resources and adequate funding, for example accessible and affordable transport and physical access to premises, which managers need to provide.

Disabled people want to be involved with the services that shape their lives and it is now rare for health and social care professionals and managers to ignore them entirely in the planning and delivery process.[34] There are, however, competing agendas and those of professionals and managers are usually given priority. Beresford et al[13] contend that user involvement schemes have become so distanced from the actual experience of service users that they have a limited impact on their day-to-day lives. This is most likely to occur when the agenda and the research instruments used in consultation have been devised by service providers without any input from service users. User involvement can easily become a side issue and this has not been helped by rapid and turbulent change within health and social services in recent years. Whereas service providers are concerned with budgets, policy and the smooth running of organisations, the concerns of disabled people are to fundamentally change, not only the services they receive, but society itself. This leads to conflict because, whereas the professional approach starts with 'the system' and how it can be adjusted, the approach of disabled people is concerned with changing the reality of their lives. Barnes and Mercer[35] relate this conflict to the underlying consumerist and democratic models of user involvement:

> On the one hand there are user led movements seeking autonomy, control and power, and on the other hand there is an agency led view of consulting with consumers about their perspectives, in line with a market economy of welfare approach.

Priestley[19] believes that true user involvement means equal partnership at the management level of organisations. Robson et al[1] note that a controlling style of management can be a strong and destructive barrier to user involvement and, conversely, a facilitatory style can be beneficial. Influential allies within the power structure can enhance the potential of users to influence decisions as can external groups such as researchers and disabled people's organisations. Robson *et al*[1] point out the need for a stable and committed staff who will assist in taking user involvement initiatives forward. They note that user involvement initiatives can be slowed down or stopped if the turnover of staff in organisations is high. The amount of time and support managers and professionals can give will, in turn, depend on how well they are supported. Priestley[19] states that:

> Effective user involvement requires a strong political commitment at the 'top' of the provider or purchaser organisation. The commitment needs to be a contractual requirement for staff at all levels.

Evans and Carmichael[36] are particularly critical of the widespread use of public meetings in user involvement initiatives. They argue:

> To engage in public meetings … demands, on the whole, familiarity and confidence with the normal style, format and language of these meetings. In addition very practical issues of physical access, transport, interpreters, signers, personal assistance and so on must be addressed by social and health services if disabled people are to be enabled to take part in consultation meetings.

'Knowledge is power' but all too often accessible information is lacking. Information needs to be accessible to all disabled people, regardless of impairment, if user involvement is to succeed. This may include information in Braille, in pictorial form, or on audiotape. Disabled people, like all people, also need background information in order to participate meaningfully.[37] Disabled people, however, face numerous barriers to accessing information and relevant services, and are consequently marginalised in any strategies for service user involvement. Being unable to access information is, for instance, a problem faced in all areas of life by visually impaired people, with potentially hazardous consequences of unreadable notices and loss of privacy when documents are unreadable by the intended recipient. The report prepared by Vale[38] provides what it calls well documented examples for this topic. For instance, appointment letters continue to be sent out in standard-size print even by many hospital eye clinics, and only one third of NHS hospitals offer general patient information in large print.

Likewise, Pound and Hewitt[39] point out the ways in which people with language impairments have been excluded from having an influence in health and social care services. They state:

> It is easy to take for granted the power of language. Language is not just the means of communicating with each other, it is the means of forming and refining ideas. It is the medium of understanding, questioning and developing thoughts and discussion. It is the means of being included, having a voice and exercising influence…
>
> Communication access is a poorly understood concept that offers intriguing challenges to all concerned with inclusionary practice. Moving beyond tokenism places significant resource and training demands on people and environments.

The pace of work can be exclusionary to many disabled people.[9] Visually impaired people, for example, may need more time to read documents and people with learning difficulties may need help in understanding concepts. Referring to people with communication impairments, Pound and Hewitt[39] argue:

The issue of time may far outweigh the relatively straightforward challenge to adapt the physical or spatial environment. The rapid rhythm and tempo of everyday life make few allowances for a calmer, slower, more deliberate form of interpersonal communication. For people with communication disabilities the slower tempo is not a choice but the only accessible pace.

Disabled people have frequently been disempowered by previous experiences, for example time spent in institutions, and need time, support and resources to build up sufficient confidence to participate fully.[40] Carmichael[12] found that consciousness raising and empowerment were very important to the disabled people in her study when seeking to influence services and Bewley and Glendinning[25] found that preliminary work with service users is frequently required before consultation can begin. If professional and managerial practice is poor with regard to user involvement this can further disempower disabled people. Carr[9] concludes from her review of the literature on user involvement that:

> If organisations are serious about listening to users, they also need to be prepared to make radical changes of approach in order to take on board what people are saying and address this in mainstream services.

As Connelly and Seden[41] advise:

> When planning the structure of services to be delivered to a diverse range of people, it is important to find service users who represent that range of diversity.

They go on to suggest that issues can arise such as whether a person with one type of impairment can represent someone with a different impairment.

Disabled people are often challenged about being unrepresentative when they express their views or when they attempt to speak on behalf of other disabled people. Evans and Carmichael[36] state that:

> Representatives from organisations of disabled people, including self-advocacy groups, were sometimes dismissed by social and health service officers as being unrepresentative of users because they appeared to be too articulate to be 'real' users.

Similarly Brown[18] notes that,

> Users who represent the movement may not be representative in the sense of being 'typical'... this may be used to challenge the legitimacy of their position in speaking for others.

Beresford and Campbell[42] believe that the emphasis by health and social care workers on the representativeness of disabled people is a way of maintaining their power base. Managers and professionals sometimes use lone disabled people from the workforce to represent other disabled people without any recognition of the conflict this position puts disabled people in.[36] 'Carers' are also asked to represent disabled people especially people with learning difficulties or those who cannot speak English.[25] Furthermore disabled people are sometimes used in a tokenistic way, for example having just one disabled person on a committee where, in effect, they have little or no power although the service may be seen to be 'doing what it has to do'. Drake[17] believes that consultation can be used as a 'sop' to offset political protest. Mercer[8] asserts that:

Too often user participation in public service provision has turned out to be little more than cosmetic.

Beresford and Campbell[42] believe that managers and professionals, who follow such practices, are in no position to criticise the representativeness of disabled people. They state:

> Questions about the mandate of disabled people and service users ignore or deny the validity of the large and growing number of democratically constituted and controlled local, regional, national and international disabled people's, services users and self-advocacy groups and organisations to which they belong and which they are elected or chosen to represent.

They go on to explain that while service professionals and managers have a representative system of democracy, disabled people's organisations have a participatory model of democracy which is characterised by consensus decision making.

A common complaint that disabled people have when they take part in user involvement initiatives is the lack of feedback they receive from managers about the impact of consultation.[25] Carr[9] states that:

> Lack of feedback can result in frustration and cynicism about the practise of service user participation as well as potential disengagement from the process altogether.

Users need a high level of involvement in order to influence services.

It is often the case that insights from users are not translated into practice by professionals and managers. Motivation can be quickly lost if their input has no effect.[13] Carr[9] speaks of 'consultation fatigue' among disabled people and Robson et al[1] note that there is sometimes a level of seniority above which service users are not permitted to go. Beresford et al[13] urge professionals to take disabled people seriously in order to move forward.

> Until service users have a sense of and confidence in the validity of the contribution they have to make, it will be difficult to establish relationships of trust with professionals and to work together on a basis of mutual respect.

Disabled people are becoming more selective in deciding when, how and to whom they will give their time, effort and views and are formulating 'rules of engagement' to be followed when their opinions are sought.[12]

Conclusion

This chapter concludes by bringing together the major factors necessary for successful user involvement among disabled people according to key workers in the field.

First, Connelly and Seden[41] offer the following summary of the possible implications of service user involvement for management:

> There are plenty of obstacles to meaningful, embedded service user consultation and involvement, not least of which is a tokenistic and mechanistic approach to the process without real commitment. There is no single service user voice, just as there is no single professional voice.

Management responses need to be flexible and informed by service users within the context of the service. The involvement of service users in interview processes, for example, may take longer to achieve in a large public sector bureaucracy than in a service user-controlled project.

Drawing on a range of research studies and reports, they also suggest that the management of developments in service user involvement needs attention to a number of factors which are summarised:

1 there is a need for support arrangements, including mentoring and training, particularly for people who have little or no experience of involvement in the planning and delivery of services
2 consideration needs to be given to the possibility of payment (or recompense) to users for their time and work in involvement
3 similarly expenses of any kind, such as that for travel or translators, need to be paid in full.

Evans[40] has made recommendations for user involvement with disabled people (see Box 7.1).

Box 7.1 Key principles for informing user involvement with disabled people. Adapted from Evans.[40]

1 The underpinning of the social model of disability.
2 User-led community development work.
3 Valuing user expertise.
4 Working with allies.
5 Building on existing user initiatives.
6 Changing from 'knowing best' to enabling users.
7 Bottom-up change.
8 'Riddling the system' with user involvement.
9 Embarking on a journey of exploration.
10 Working in bite sized chunks.

With regard to point ten she states:

It is all too easy to get so overwhelmed by wanting to change the world that one fails to get started. Faced with the conservative nature of social services and health bureaucracies even the small changes user organisations make need to be recognised and celebrated.

Gibbs and Priestley[43] developed a user involvement checklist (see Box 7.2).

Box 7.2 User involvement checklist. Adapted from Gibbs and Priestley.[43]

• Does your organisation want to increase user power?
• Are your staff required to demonstrate a commitment to user involvement?
• If you impose limits on user power do you make these clear to everyone?
• Are your environments, processes and information accessible to disabled people?

- Do you involve disabled people's organisations as well as individual users?
- Do disabled people control your user involvement process?
- Do disabled people control your user involvement agenda for consultation issues?
- Do you provide user representatives with the same support systems as staff representatives?
- Do you communicate the outcomes of disabled people's involvement back to them?
- Has your organisation ever made changes against its will because disabled people wanted you to?

Beresford and Croft[7] provide six elements which they believe contribute to successful user involvement:

1 the resourcing of user led organisations
2 systematic and central involvement of users in professional training
3 self-definition of need and design of services by service users
4 equal access and opportunities for disabled service users
5 user-led standard setting and definition of outcomes in policy and practice
6 user led monitoring and evaluation of provision.

Successful user involvement is not easy not least because disabled people are a diverse and heterogeneous group and as Bewley and Glendinning[25] put it:

> To expect that consultation will reveal a single common view is an illusion...

These tensions can be made worse if more than one group of users are involved who have different ideologies and historical roots, for example disabled people and 'carers' where 'carers' usually have more power. However, Carr[9] points out that user involvement can be tremendously beneficial to organisations as it provides:

> A unique opportunity for organisations to develop and transform through critical enquiry with service users.

Robson *et al*[1] make the point that:

> When user involvement is second nature to enough people in an organisation it becomes 'the way we do things round here' and in a sense does not seek to exist as a separate or optional activity.

Turning specifically to management and management culture, it is possible to suggest a number of crucial factors with regard to user involvement. First, the development of service user involvement needs to be given presidency and promoted across a management team, including senior managers. Second, managers need to communicate directly with service users and not through intermediaries. Third, particularly in multi-professional teams and collaboration across service boundaries; joint working will be required to facilitate collaboration and co-operation.

Managers need to develop a culture in which power can be shared. The development of service user involvement also needs to be managed within a continuous process of change, requiring flexibility and ongoing monitoring which also involves service users. Finally, turning to the management of budgeting issues, it is clear that service user involvement needs to be understood in the broadest context. In managing care, for instance, 'Best Value' – a process initiated by government to achieve efficient and effective social services through benchmarking, consultation and competition – affects managers in all settings and is a process that requires the ability to address notions of quality and cost. Gallop[44] states:

> The 'old' attitude of 'we know best' had, if nothing else, the advantage of making judgement more straightforward. Its considerable disadvantage was that it created services based on paternalism, where the provider, not the user, defined quality. Similarly, judgements made solely on cost will not meet the Best Value test either … The commitment to embrace more than one perspective opens up possibilities for more creative service development. Real partnership with service users in particular increases the likelihood of a Best Value (and best value) outcome.

Disabled people are becoming empowered within society and are no longer prepared to have decisions made on their behalf. It is the challenge of managers and professionals in health and social care to ensure, not only that the involvement of disabled people is possible, but that it is extensive, meaningful and translated into practice with positive outcomes for their lives.

References

1 Robson P, Begum N, Locke M. *Developing User Involvement*. Bristol: Policy Press; 2003.
2 Croft S, Beresford P. Service Users' Perspectives. In: Davies M, editor. *Companion to Social Work*. 2nd ed. Oxford: Blackwell; 2002.
3 Hughes G, Lewis G. *Unsettling Welfare: the reconstruction of social policy*. London: Routledge; 1996.
4 Furgusson R, Hughes G, Neal S. Welfare: from security to responsibility? In: Hughes G, Furgusson R, editors. *Ordering Lives: family, work and welfare*. 2nd ed. London: Routledge; 2004.
5 Act of Parliament. Children's Act. London: The Stationery Office; 1989.
6 Act of Parliament. The National Health Service and Community Care Act. London: The Stationery Office; 1990.
7 Beresford P, Croft S. User Involvement. In: Davies M, editor. *The Blackwell Encyclopaedia of Social Work*. Oxford: Blackwell; 2000.
8 Mercer G. User-Led Organisations: facilitation independent living. In: Swain J, French S, Barnes C, *et al*, editors. *Disabling Barriers – enabling environments*. 2nd ed. London: Sage; 2004.
9 Carr S. *Has Service User Involvement Made a Difference to Social Care Services?* London: Social Institute for Excellence; 2004.
10 O'Sullivan T. Decision Making in Social Work. In: Davies M, editor. *The Blackwell Encyclopaedia of Social Work*. Oxford: Blackwell Publishers; 2000.
11 Department of Health. Reforming the Mental Health Act: Part 1 The New Legal Framework. London: The Stationery Office; 2000.
12 Carmichael A. The social model, the emancipatory paradigm and user involvement. In: Barnes C, Mercer G, editors. *Implementing the Social Model of Disability: theory and research*. Leeds: The Disability Press; 2004.

13 Beresford P, Croft S, Evans C, *et al*. Quality in personal social services: the developing role of user involvement in the UK. In: Evans A, Haverinen K, Leichsering K, *et al*. editors. *Developing Quality in Personal Social Services*. Aldershot: Ashgate; 1997.

14 Braye S. Participation and involvement in social care: an overview. In: Kemshall H, Littlechild R, editors. *User Involvement and Participation in Social Care*. London: Jessica Kingsley; 2000.

15 Campbell J, Oliver M. *Disability Policies: understanding our past, changing our future*. London: Routledge; 1996.

16 Barton L. The disability movement: some observations. In: Swain J, French S, Barnes C, *et al*. editors. *Disabling Barriers – enabling environments*. 2nd ed. London: Sage; 2004.

17 Drake R. *Understanding Disability Policies*. Basingstoke: Macmillan; 1996.

18 Brown H. Challenges from Service Users. In: Brechin A, Brown H, Ely M. editors. *Critical Practice in Health and Social Care*. London: Sage; 2000.

19 Priestley M. *Disability Politics and Community Care*. London: Jessica Kingsley; 1999.

20 Act of Parliament. Disability Discrimination Act. London: The Stationery Office; 1995.

21 Department for Constitutional Affairs. Study Guide on Human Rights Act 1998. 2nd ed. October 2002.

22 Act of Parliament. Disability Rights Commission Act. London: The Stationery Office; 1999.

23 European Convention of Human Rights. Available at: shttp://www.hri.org/docs/ECHR50.html.

24 Goss S, Miller C. *From Margin to Mainstream: developing user and carer-centred community care*. York: Joseph Rowntree Foundation; 1995.

25 Bewley C, Glendinning C. *Involving Disabled People in Community Care Planning*. York: Joseph Rowntree Foundation; 1994.

26 Atkin C, French S, Vernon A. Health care for people from ethnic minority groups. In: French S, Sim J, editors. *Physiotherapy: a psychosocial approach*. 3rd ed. Oxford: Butterworth-Heinemann; 2004.

27 Banton M, Singh G. Race, disability and oppression. In: Swain J, French S, Barnes C, *et al*. editors. *Disabling Barriers – enabling environments*. 2nd ed. London: Sage; 2004.

28 Swain J, French S. Researching Together: a participatory approach. In: French S, Sim J, editors. *Physiotherapy: a psychosocial approach*. Oxford: Butterworth-Heinemann; 2004.

29 Faulkner A, Layzell S. *Strategies for Living: a report of user-led research intro people's strategies for living with mental distress*. London: Mental Health Foundation; 2000.

30 Evans C, Fisher J. Collaborative evaluation with service users. In: Shaw I, Lishman J, editors. *Evaluation and Social Work Practice*. London: Sage; 1999.

31 French S, Swain J. The relationship between disabled people and health and welfare professionals. In: Albrecht G, Seelman K, Bury M, editors. *Handbook of Disability Studies*. London: Sage; 2001.

32 Goble C. Dependence, independence and normality. In: Swain J, French S, Barnes C, *et al*, editors. *Disabling Barriers – enabling environments*. 2nd ed. London: Sage; 2004.

33 Finkelstein V. Modernising services? In: Swain J, French S, Barnes C, *et al*, editors. *Disabling Barriers – enabling environments*. 2nd ed. London: Sage; 2004.

34 Beresford P, Croft S, Evans C, *et al*. Quality in personal social services: the developing role of user involvement in the UK. In: Davies C, Finlay L, Bullman A, editors. *Changing Practice in Health and Social Care*. London: Sage; 2000.

35 Barnes C, Mercer G. *Disability*. Cambridge: Polity Press; 2003.

36 Evans C, Carmichael A, members of the Direct Payment Best Value Project Group of Wiltshire and Swindon Users' Network. *Users' Best Value: a guide to user involvement good practice in Best Value Reviews*. York: Joseph Rowntree Foundation; 2002.

37 Evans C. From those who know: the role of service users. In: Hanvey C, Philpot T, editors. *Sweet Charity: the role and workings of voluntary organisations*. London: Routledge; 1996.

38 Vale D. *Improving Lives: priorities in health social care for blind and partially sighted people*. On behalf of the Improving Lives Coalition by the Royal National Institute for the Blind. London: RNIB; 2001.

39 Pound C, Hewitt A. Communication barriers: building access and identity. In: Swain J, French S, Barnes C, *et al.* editors. *Disabling Barriers – enabling environments*. 2nd ed. London: Sage; 2004.

40 Evans C. Gaining our voice: the development patterns of good practice in user involvement. *Managing Community Care*. 1999; **7**(2): 7–13.

41 Connelly N, Seden J. What service users say about services: the implications for managers. In: Henderson J, Atkinson D, editors. *Managing Care in Context*. London: Routledge; 2003.

42 Beresford P, Campbell J. Disabled people, service users, user involvement and representation. *Disability and Society*.1994; **9**(3): 315–25.

43 Gibbs D, Priestley M. The social model and user involvement. In: Walker B editor. *Disability Rights: a symposium of the European regions*. Headley, Hampshire: Hampshire Coalition of Disabled People; 1996.

44 Gallop L. Managing budgets and giving best value. In: Seden J, Reynolds J, editors. *Managing Care In Practice*. London: Sage; 2003.

Chapter 8

Corporate governance and the health professional

Tove Steen Sørensen-Bentham

Corporate governance has become increasingly important throughout society, since effective governance is the cornerstone of well-managed organisations whether they are in the public, private or voluntary sectors. Audit Commission 2005[1]

Governance

Corporate governance lays down the 'rules' which organisations operate within. The healthcare manager needs to understand this framework in order to manage services in accord with legislative and other requirements. Failure to comprehend this area of management may leave the manager open to significant risk and the organisation subject to criticism and censure.

The principles of governance for the public services are based on models which were designed for the private sector where corporate governance is seen as: the way in which companies are directed and controlled. Based on the Cadbury definition[2] the Organisation for Economic Co-operation and Development (OECD) has drawn up its own principles of corporate governance and states that:

> Good corporate governance involves a set of relationships between a company's management, its board, its shareholders and other stakeholders. Corporate governance also provides the structure through which the objectives of the company are set, and the means of attaining those objectives and monitoring performance.[3]

However, currently there is not a single accepted definition or model of good corporate governance[4] despite major corporate failures in recent years such as Enron and World.com. These organisational collapses have highlighted the devastating impact of weak governance systems and have at an international level raised the importance of ensuring strong governance arrangements.

Public service governance principles have been strongly influenced by a number of reports in the UK into governance in the private sector such as Cadbury,[2] Hampel,[5] Turnbull,[6] Smith,[7] and Higgs.[8] These reports have resulted in 'The Combined Code: Principles of Good Governance and Code of Best Practice'[9]. Based on the governance development within the private sector and various reports from the Audit Commission,[1,10,11] over the last decade a debate about the concept for corporate governance in the public sector has taken place, especially during the last few years, culminating in the establishment in 2004 of an

Independent Commission for Good Governance in Public Services to develop a common standard of governance for all public services. The Independent Commission[12] identified six principles of good governance which it believed were common to all public service organisations and partnerships using public money.

1 Good governance means focusing on the organisation's purpose and on outcomes for citizens and service users.
2 Good governance means performing effectively in clearly defined functions and roles.
3 Good governance means promoting values for the whole organisation and demonstrating the values of good governance through behaviour.
4 Good governance means taking informed, transparent decisions and managing risk.
5 Good governance means developing the capacity and capability of the governing body to be effective.
6 Good governance means engaging stakeholders and making accountability real.

Despite the establishment of these governance principles for all public services, including a lot of services delivered by the voluntary and community services, a separate code of good governance for the voluntary and community sector was subsequently developed by a number of voluntary sector infrastructure bodies and the Charity Commission[13] as this sector seems to be of the view that the good governance standards for public services are not suitable for them but for the public sector only. This raises the debate about which sets of governance principles should be applied for services provided by the voluntary sector on behalf of the public sector. These are services which normally are covered by the term 'public services'.

Just as the private sector – despite governance codes and principles – has not got a common definition of corporate governance, so is it the case for the public services. Given this lack of clarity, it might be most relevant for public service organisations to apply the governance definition provided by the Audit Commission as this body provides the regulatory framework for governance in the public services in practice:[10]

> The framework of accountability to users, stakeholders and the wider community, within which organisations take decisions, and lead and control their functions, to achieve their objectives.

This definition together with the good governance principles defined by the Independent Commission[12] and the Association of Chief Executives of the Voluntary Organisations (ACEVO)[13] are all building on the code of conduct established by the Nolan Report[14] which defined the principles of governance for people in public office to be as shown in Box 8.1.

Surprisingly, the Nolan principles have not been updated since the first report by the Nolan Committee despite the changes that have taken place in the public services and the increased emphasis on delivering services appropriate for the service users. Other standards which, especially in an increasingly complex political, economic, legislative and central versus local context, should be considered as equally relevant for ensuring good governance in public office are transparency, fairness and accessibility.

Box 8.1 The seven principles of public life.

1 **Selflessness**. Holders of public office should take decisions solely in terms of the public interest. They should not do so in order to gain financial or other material benefits for themselves, their family, or their friends.

2 **Integrity.** Holders of public office should not place themselves under any financial or other obligation to outside individuals or organisations that might influence them in the performance of their official duties.

3 **Objectivity**. In carrying out public office, including making public appointments, awarding contracts, or recommending individuals for rewards and benefits, holders of public office should make choices on merit.

4 **Accountability.** Holders of public office are accountable for their decisions and actions to the public and must submit themselves to whatever scrutiny is appropriate to their office.

5 **Openness**. Holders of public office should be as open as possible about all the decisions and actions that they take. They should give reasons for their decisions and restrict information only when the wider public interest clearly demands.

6 **Honesty.** Holders of public office have a duty to declare any private interest relating to their public duties and to take steps to resolve any conflicts arising in any way that protects the public interest.

7 **Leadership.** Holders of public office should promote and support these principles by leadership and example.

Both Nolan and the Independent Commission principles are primarily aimed at ensuring public trust and confidence in the decision making processes through the involvement of service users and the wider public and through the clarity of those processes.

All publicly funded organisations are responsible for ensuring that the services provided are appropriate for the needs of the service users and that resources are utilised in the most effective and efficient way. One of the underpinning principles for ensuring this is by establishing clear governance arrangement and the way of demonstrating this is through the public accountability arrangements. Governance and accountability is thus intertwined.

The principles of public accountability together with national standards are explicitly mentioned in the Government's principles of public service reforms. Scrivens[15] argues that greater emphasis on local accountability is required if the Government is delivering the public service reforms though a devolution of decision making in order to ensure that services are both meeting the needs of the service users and are provided appropriately and consistently across the country.

The debate in the private sector concerning the impact of governance arrangements on innovation in business practice has also been raised by public service organisations which, at times, find it difficult to find solutions to complex service user needs within a requirement of having to demonstrate accountability and probity in the use of public resources.

The details of the governance arrangements are normally found in the organisation's Code of Conduct and its system of internal controls which in the NHS covers the three elements of financial, organisational and clinical control. The increasing requirement for organisations to pay greater attention to the internal control and risk management systems led to the formation of the Turnbull Committee which, in its 1999 report, aimed at providing organisations with guidance on how to develop and maintain systems of internal control.[4]

All NHS bodies are expected to adhere to the accounting standards set out by the Government internal Audit Standards and these provide a framework for good accounting practices against which the individual organisation's audited accounts are assessed by both internal and external auditors for compliance and robustness. The NHS Code of Conduct and Accountability sets out the overall responsibilities and requirement for financial control for NHS organisations and the DH issues specific guidance to its organisations in health services circulars. It is the overall responsibility of the Board to ensure that proper systems of internal control are in place. However, chief executives of NHS Trusts are the designated accountable officers on all financial matters including performance. In practice the chief executive delegates the day-to-day operational responsibility for the financial matters to the director of finance.

It is the clear responsibility of the Board to review the effectiveness of all internal controls including the risk management systems. The activities of the audit and the risk management committees support the Board receiving the appropriate level of assurance. The financial controls are normally specified in the organisation's standing financial instructions and it is the responsibility of the NHS Board to formally adopt these. In order to demonstrate how the Boards have received the required level of assurance that the internal controls are in place, all NHS Boards are now required to publish an annual assurance statement also called the 'Statement of Internal Controls', which is signed off by the organisation's chief executive on behalf of the Board. Each individual NHS Board is therefore responsible for ensuring an effective system of corporate governance through its adoption of Standards of Business Conducts, Standing Financial Instruction, Standing Orders and Scheme of Delegation. These cover a very diverse range of issues from declaration of interest, fraud and corruption, hospitality, sponsorship, charitable funds, freedom of information, Caldicott Guardian scheme and so on. A broad range of guidance is available from both the Department of Health and the NHS Appointment Commission about the responsibilities of the Board.

Good corporate governance is not just about setting up the formal system; often called the 'hard' factors, such as robust systems and processes, which can too easily be used against a 'tick-box' exercise for compliance. The need to avoid such a superficial approach was stressed by the Hampel Report[5] which stated:

> Good corporate governance is not just a matter of prescribing particular corporate structures and complying with a number of hard and fast rules. There is a need for broad principles … There is another problem with box ticking. It can be seized on as an easier option than the diligent pursuit of corporate governance objectives. It would then not be difficult for lazy or unscrupulous directors – or shareholders – to arrange matters so that the letter of every governance rule was complied with but not the substance. It

might even be possible for the next disaster to emerge in a company with, on paper, a 100% record of compliance. The true safeguard for good corporate governance lies in the application of informed and independent judgement by experienced and qualified individuals – executive and non-executive directors, shareholders and auditors.

Good governance should therefore also encompass the less tangible aspects of organisations which can be described as the 'softer' characteristics. These include effective leadership and high standards of individual behaviour as well as within the organisational culture as a whole. In order for organisations to ensure strong governance systems they will need to establish a strong internal organisational culture based on identified and agreed governance principles. They also need to ensure organisational capability and ability to carry out effective 'horizon scanning' of the external environment in order to position the organisation optimally with regard to its strategic objectives. The Audit Commission[10] found that this internal combination of 'hard' and 'soft' characteristics involves:

- leadership that establishes a vision for organisations, generates clarity about strategy and objectives, roles and responsibilities, and fosters professional relationships
- culture based on openness and honesty, in which decisions and behaviours can be challenged and accountability is clear
- accountability through systems and processes, such as risk management, financial management, performance management and internal controls. They must be robust and produce reliable information to enable better decisions to be reached about what needs to be done in order to achieve objectives
- external focus on the needs of service users and the public, reflecting diverse views in decision making, producing greater ownership among stakeholders and maintaining clarity of purpose.

The overall responsibility for governance in organisations rests with the governing body, which in NHS organisations is the Board. The Board can have a varying number of members which includes both executive and non-executive directors. The main function of an NHS Board and of an organisation's governance arrangement is thus to ensure that the organisation can achieve its overall objectives set out in its strategy, can deliver its planned services to its service users to a high standard of quality and that all its activities are performed effectively and efficiently thereby creating 'public value' for its community.

Absence of good governance

The absence of proper governance structures leaves organisations at greater risk of failure or being ineffective and inefficient. Amongst the most common risks to partnership working in the public services identified by the Audit Commission[11] are:

- failure to understand the extent of their involvement in partnerships, or its implications, including their financial and legal liabilities
- absent or insufficient corporate criteria to enable public bodies to assess whether to form a partnership or participate in one, what the appropriate level of involvement should be and what resources to invest

- insufficient thought given to planning an exit strategy
- lack of clarity on insurable risk, such as indemnity cover for partner members or public liability
- lack of formal systems for recording conflicts of interests or for assessing the risks of funding proposals.

Having analysed a number of reports examining serious public service failures in recent years the Audit Commission[10] identified a number of common themes relating to governance. These were:

- poor quality or absence of leadership
- poor decision making and decision-making processes
- inadequate systems and processes, such as performance management
- lack of clarity in roles, responsibilities and activities creating poor accountability
- poor working relationships and dysfunctional behaviours
- an insular organisational culture and poor focus on community and user needs
- inadequate contingency plans or risk management strategies to deal with worst-case scenarios.

The crucial element in this identification of common denominators for governance failures is that service failures rarely occur due to one of these themes being present but are caused by a combination of factors not necessarily only including these. Organisations with weak governance systems might therefore be characterised by the existence of one or more of these themes even though the organisations have not yet experienced a serious service failure. However, for those organisations there is a constant latent danger that a serious failure will occur.

The cost of not having appropriate governance systems in place is not only the financial cost to the organisation by having to address the identified short comings, for example having to establish a strong and appropriate governance structure and culture. The greatest loss is to the service users who have not received the services they reasonably could expect – and to society as a whole – as trust in the public service is closely linked to the ability of the service to deliver the right service, to the right individuals, at the right time and at the right price. Whilst trust takes a long time to be earned it takes far less for trust to be lost. Lack of good governance can therefore lead to serious damage to reputation and credibility not just to an individual organisation but by association to a whole sector.

Clinical governance

In addition to ensuring proper systems of corporate governance, NHS organisations have an additional responsibility for ensuring clinical governance. This is the central element of the framework through which NHS organisations are accountable for continuously improving the quality of their services that supports the delivery of quality of services.[16] Scally and Donaldson[17] comment:

> Clinical governance is a system through which NHS organisations are accountable for continuously improving the quality of their services and safeguarding high standards of care by creating an environment in which excellence in clinical care will flourish.

'The New NHS Modern and Dependable' White Paper[18] together with 'A First Class Service'[16] and supported by the NHS Plan[19] established the Government quality agenda as a driving force for the development of healthcare.

'Clinical Governance: in the New NHS'[20] established the need to focus on the activities involved in delivering high quality care to patients by stating:

> It will mean the creation of a systematic set of mechanisms that will support staff and develop all health organisations to deliver a new approach to quality.

Amongst the many reasons given regarding the need for a comprehensive quality drive in the NHS are:

- NHS not meeting modern expectation of high quality patient care
- well published cases of untoward incidents and mis-management
- postcode lottery
- unacceptable variance in performance
- slow introduction of evidence-based practice
- inequality in patient outcomes, waiting times and so on.

Whilst people working in the NHS strive to achieve good quality care, it is acknowledged that this effort sometimes falls short of the aspirations. Clinical governance is therefore intended to be an open and helpful process, embracing all members of clinical teams and supporting those who are falling behind in delivering best care. It aims to identify poor performance and, in part, tackle all issues causing poor performance although it is, at times, also used alongside other contractual and regulatory methods.

The main components of clinical governance are:

- clear lines of responsibility and accountability for the overall quality of clinical care
- a comprehensive programme of quality improvement systems (including clinical audit, supporting and applying evidence-based practice, implementing clinical standards and guidelines, workforce planning and development)
- education and training plans
- clear policies aimed at managing risk
- integrated procedures for all professional groups to identify and remedy poor performance.

Healthcare organisations are expected to deliver high quality services through clinical governance underpinned by modernised professional self-regulation and extended life-long learning.[21] The quality concept is supported by standards given by standards for services and treatments by the National Services Frameworks (NSFs)[22] and the National Institute for Health and Clinical Excellence (NICE).

The independent monitoring and promoting of improvement in the quality of healthcare and public health in England and Wales is the responsibility of the Commission for Healthcare Audit and Inspection (CHAI) which was formed by the Health and Social Care (Community Health and Standards) Act 2003 and launched in 2004 as a successor body to the Commission for Health Improvement (CHI). It has also taken over some responsibilities from other organisations. These include the private and voluntary healthcare functions of the National Care Standards Commission covering elements of the Audit Commission's work which relate to efficiency, effectiveness and economy of healthcare.

CHAI has been given the following main responsibilities:[23]

Box 8.2 Main responsibilities of CHAI.

- **Inspect**: to inspect the quality and value for money of healthcare and public health
- **Inform**: to equip patients and the public with the best possible information about the provision of healthcare
- **Improve**: to promote improvements in healthcare and public health

---

CHAI is also responsible for reviewing the performance of each local NHS organisation and awarding an annual rating of that organisation based on a set of core and developmental standards, which were identified in 2005/2006 DoH Standards for Better Health 2004.[24] The core standards are those that all NHS organisations in England now should be achieving. Developmental standards are those of good practice that they should be aiming to achieve in the future.

The standards cover seven domains:

1 safety
2 clinical and cost effectiveness
3 governance
4 patient focus
5 accessible and responsive care
6 care environment and amenities
7 public health.

The standards for health take into account the NSFs, which set standards of provision in areas of care that have a high priority, and the guidance issued by NICE.

The core standard on governance includes principles of sound clinical and corporate governance including the responsibility for ensuring compliance with the requirement of research governance (Core standard C12) as set out in the Research Governance Framework for Health and Social Care.[25]

The Research Governance Framework establishes that the primary consideration of any research study must be the 'dignity, rights, safety and well being of participants in NHS related research'. Any research proposal will need approval from the local Research Ethics Committee, whilst audits and evaluation of services might not require this. The difference between research, clinical audits and service evaluation might at times be difficult to discern. However, most management studies are aimed at improving the current quality of services by evaluating the services delivered against the organisational aims and objectives and national benchmarking rather than involving any data relating to service users. Although this work does not always require approval from the local Research Ethics Committee, it is advisable always to seek permission from the Trust involved.

Within individual organisations the continuous quality agenda requires organisations to focus on the implementation and management of and adherence to processes such as monitoring of activities against targets, clinical audits, risk management, adverse incident reporting, complaints, evidence-based practice and service user involvement.

The chief executive and the Board within NHS organisations are ultimately responsible for both corporate and clinical governance. However, for clinical governance to be effective it requires input from all clinical professionals who are individually accountable for their professional practices. Although the term 'clinical governance' infers a reference solely to clinical activities it can be argued that clinical governance is not a responsibility reserved for clinical professionals. As clinical governance is about quality of services in all of its various components, it could be argued that it should be a responsibility for everyone working in the NHS. In order to ensure the effective delivery of continuous quality improvement within NHS organisations it is thus important that each individual has a clear understanding of the concept of quality and that this quality concept is developed together with and shared by the service users and is ingrained within the organisational culture.

Any successful quality agenda requires that quality is an issue that concerns everyone and that the Boards and senior management within the NHS provide constant leadership to ensure successfully that a shared definition of quality exists and that quality is implemented, monitored and accounted for. Quality initiatives need to permeate the organisations through a vertical top-down and bottom-up approach supplemented by a horizontal quality approach that reaches out to partner organisations whether they are in other parts of the NHS, in the not-for-profit or the private sector.

Governance in joint working across the public services

With the advent of the modernisation agenda for the public services since the Labour Government took office in 1997, service users and the local communities have increasingly become central to the strategic planning process for public service organisations. However, since the pathways for delivering effective user-centred care often affect more than one public service organisation there has been both a statutory requirement and a political pressure towards partnership and other forms of joint working across statutory, voluntary and independent sector organisations and more recently, also with private sector companies.

Partnership working has grown rapidly, encouraged by legislation that removed previous barriers and granted new powers to organisations to work collaboratively through pooling budgets, agreeing lead commissioning arrangements and delivering integrated services. Governance is particularly important in partnership arrangements where lines of accountability can be complex and/or unclear as services are no longer provided within a single organisational hierarchical structure. Where activity is integrated across agencies, it is particularly important that the partnership agreement includes transparent decision making processes together with clarity about executive authority, accountability and the effective scrutiny of performance. Research into partnerships in the UK has identified that problems with governance arise due to the very structure of partnerships which are designed around vertical and horizontal integration in policy implementation instead of around democratic needs.[26]

To ensure proper accountability for partnership activity, the governance arrangements need to be clear, and should indicate the opportunity for local communities to influence their local services.

Public services, whether they be local authorities, the police service or the NHS are increasingly dependent on delivering services through partnership or other forms of joint working arrangements such as networks and strategic alliances.

The powers to enable health and local authority partners to work together more effectively came into force in 2000. These were outlined in Section 31 of the 1999 Health Act and are aimed at health bodies such as PCTs and NHS Trusts and any health related local authority service such as housing, social services, transport and leisure. The guidance on the establishment of proper governance arrangements was outlined in the advisory note to the Health Act.[27]

The partnership powers introduced were:

- pooled budgets – the ability for partners to contribute to agreed funds within a single 'pot' and for these to be spent on agreed projects for designated services
- lead commissioning – partners agree to delegate commissioning of a service to one lead organisation
- integrated provision – partners can join together staff, resources and management structures to integrate the provision of a service.

Joint working arrangements outside the 1999 Health Act can also extend across sectors in a number of different combinations such as:

- public sector – public sector joint working
- public sector – not-for-profit (third sector) joint working
- public sector – private sector joint working.

Working across sectors and with organisations adhering to different governance principles may result in lack of clarity concerning lines of accountability. The Audit Commission[11] support this:

We believe strongly that partners must reach agreement on how they will govern their collaboration. It is vital that there is clarity among partners about purpose, membership, roles and responsibilities, among other things. This agreement should be set out in formal agreements.

Where activities are integrated across agencies, it is equally important that the partnership agreement includes transparent decision making processes together with clarity about executive and delegated authority, delegation of functions, statutory responsibilities and accountability and the effective scrutiny of performance including means of measuring performance against targets and quality assurance.

Health and Social Care Joint Guidance on governance arrangements for partnerships[28] ... summarises the aims of good governance as allowing public service bodies and individuals within them to provide an account of:

- improved performance in respect of outcomes of the arrangements
- their operational objectives and priorities
- proper and efficient use of public money
- the quality of services provided.

The Audit Commission[29] argues that:

Partnership working is often expensive, as well as difficult. Many of the costs involved, particularly senior and middle managers' time, are not routinely recorded and few partnerships have precise information about the costs of their activities. Nevertheless, it is clear that the time and effort required to run the growing number of partnerships is considerable: larger authorities might now participate in as many as 50 separate arrangements with other public agencies or with the private and voluntary sectors.

If partnership working is to provide good value for money, it is essential that these costs are outweighed by the benefits achieved. It is worrying, therefore, that few partnerships have collected the sort of information that would tell them whether this is the case.

The Audit Commission[11] also asks the crucial governance question:

How do partnerships add value? Evidence that partnership working brings real benefits exists, but ... Partnership working takes up a lot of time and other resources. It can therefore extract value as well as add to it, but remarkably there is very little hard information about its impact. Not all organisations even know how many partnerships they are involved in.

Who is in charge of partnerships? The Audit Commission's work in reviewing partnerships shows ... that things can easily go wrong. A third of those working in partnerships experience problems ... These problems arise when governance and accountability are weak: leadership, decision-making, scrutiny and systems and processes such as risk management are all under-developed in partnerships.

The Audit Commission places the responsibility for governance not only at the door of public organisations involved in the partnership working but at all levels within the public sector ranging from the individual organisation to the inspecting bodies and through to central Government.

In the context of partnership working this means asking pertinent questions about the governance arrangements in place:[11]

- how do your partnership's corporate governance arrangements link to those of individual partners?
- how are decisions made?
- how are they recorded?
- who makes sure that they are acted on?
- who scrutinises them?
- to whom are they reported?

The Audit Commission issued a bulletin[30] which listed the arrangements for ensuring accountability and stresses the importance of these arrangements being clearly stated and understood by all:

- the roles and responsibilities of the accountable body and the partnership needs to be formally recorded
- there should be a memorandum that sets out clearly the responsibilities and the roles of the partnership board, the partners, the partnership executive team and the project deliverers
- decision making should always be undertaken at the right level for example strategic decisions made by the partnership board
- the partnership board should meet regularly and the meetings be conducted in accordance with agreed principles

- there should be procedures for dealing with conflicts for example complaints, disciplinary.

Based on work carried out into governance and accountability in partnerships, the Audit Commission published the document 'Bridging the Accountability Gap'[11] which identified a range of key strategic and operational principles and challenges to establishing good partnership governance. The key messages included:

1 partnerships are essential to improve some – but not all – services
2 partnerships bring risks as well as opportunities, for example who is in charge of partnerships
3 partnerships bring costs as well as benefits – how and when do partnerships add value?
4 not all partnerships engage the public effectively
5 the principles of good governance are harder to apply in partnerships.

These messages are also supported by the Health and Social Care Joint Guidance on governance arrangements for partnerships under the Health Act Section 31 that states that to ensure proper accountability for partnership activity, the governance arrangements need to be clear, and should indicate the opportunity for people to influence their local services.

Accountability

> Accountability is being 'liable to be called to account', that is to explain one's actions to others, and by inference in this context, publicly… Accountability is regarded as one of three pillars of democratic Government.[15]

In addition to the responsibility for ensuring good governance arrangement it is important for public service organisation to ensure that the same attention is paid to its accountability arrangements. Public service organisations as bodies are accountable to a range of different stakeholders for financial management, service delivery, quality, strategic direction and targets. Internally, within these organisations, the individuals are accountable to varying degrees for the activities carried out. Public accountability can take many forms from publicising strategic plans, holding decision making meetings in public, publication of annual reports including accounts and performance against targets. Internal accountability will normally be demonstrated through compliance with the internal control systems.

In the public services, accountability and responsibility are commonly used concepts, although there is at times some confusion around their use and the use of the term 'authority'.

Authority can be defined as 'the right to guide or direct the actions of others and extract from them responses that are appropriate to the attainment of an organisation's goals.'[31] This means that a person 'normally' should not be made accountable for an action, which the they do not have the authority to carry out.

Responsibility, according to the same writers, is an obligation placed upon a person who occupies a certain position within an organisation structure to perform a task, function or assignment. In a situation where manager X delegates authority down to worker Y, X remains the responsible person.

Accountability is – on the other hand – the obligation of a subordinate to report back on the discharge of their responsibilities.[31] Within the organisational context this is normally clarified in the standing orders, in job descriptions and in the schemes of delegation. Accountability is therefore seen as part of the control methods used to ensure that staff do what is necessary to achieve the organisation's objectives[15] but also necessary to ensure that the ways in which the objectives are reached are acceptable to the shareholders in a private organisation and to Government, the regulatory bodies and the public at large in public sector organisations such as the NHS. When the level of trust is low there is a tendency for calling organisations or individuals within them publicly to account whilst there are not the same demands in times of high level of trust. The importance of accountability and trust is, furthermore, clearly established as one of the underlying principles of the New NHS[18] which states that it wants 'to rebuild public confidence in the NHS as a public service accountable to patients, open to the public and shaped by their views'. However, the deepening financial deficit facing a number of NHS organisations during the last few financial years combined with the threat of hospital closures and removal of local services in order to provide better quality and more efficient service delivery has done little to rebuild public confidence. This has been further aggravated by a number of high profile serious organisational failures within the NHS as illustrated by the Bristol and Shipman Inquiries – see Chapters 8, 9 and 10 in *Managing and Leading in the Allied Health Professions* earlier in this series.

Working within and across complex or new NHS organisations can at times give cause for uncertainty with regard to accountability, responsibility and authority and it is therefore important that there is clarification within the process and procedures governing decision making.

In partnership or other joint working arrangements it is even more important that the relationships between authority, accountability and responsibility are clarified from the outset rather than when things 'go wrong'. Amongst the kind of questions which might usefully be asked are listed in Box 8.3:

Box 8.3 Partnership working questions.

- Accountability - Accountable to whom? Each partner retains its own accountability arrangement but for what?
- Accountability for joint decisions – scope and details?
- Who decides the membership of and power distribution within a partnership?
- What mandates do members bring with them from their partner organisations?
- How are decisions made about the size of the budgets to be allocated to partnership schemes, or about the eligible (and ineligible) target user group?
- What decisions can be made by the partnership without the prior approval of senior managers from the partner organisations? Degree of delegated authority and delegation of functions.
- Is the scope of the decision making so wide that it raises questions about the accountability of the partnership, or so narrow that it constrains innovation?

- Who supervises/regulates the professional behaviour within a partnership?
- Who deals with joint staff grievances or disciplinaries?
- Who is accountable for complaints by users over joint services?
- Which accountable arrangement needs to be in place if part of the joint service is delivered by a 'third' party e.g. a private or voluntary organisation?
- Are the governance arrangements written down, fully understood and agreed by all partners?

Governance for the future public services

Governance for the public services is a very complex and changing concept and it has a number of main ingredients. Proper financial management is but one, alongside risk management, Code of Conduct including leadership and organisational culture, partnership working, accountability and the establishment of trust. Whilst it is possible to manage effectively some aspects of governance such as finance and risks, other aspects are not within the power of the organisation to the same degree. The behaviour of individuals within public sector organisations such as the NHS can be influenced by Codes of Conduct but underlying organisational cultures might work against these just as public confidence and trust is often more affected by the media coverage of serious incidents than by evidence-based decisions. It is therefore vital for managers and professionals to realise that whilst it can take years to build public trust and confidence in public services it can take only a second to lose it. However, by building services and organisations around sound governance structures and by incorporating and strengthening the underpinning conduct for delivering services with accountability, organisations stand a greater change of not failing but of profiting from the pressures of ever increasing demands for better, more effective and efficient services.

Another issue of concern for the robustness and quality of governance arrangements in the future is the lack of integration between the various governance systems and potential for overlap and duplication. The result of this for NHS organisations[32] is that Boards become unfocused, as separate governance streams presented to the boards are either too general or too complex to be useful for the Boards to exercise their scrutiny role. By integrating governance, not only should Boards benefit, but also patients, as it is in their interests that quality of services are better assured. A handbook for NHS Boards[33] has been issued to assist with the integration of governance within NHS organisations. The development in the NHS is not just about the health services but has significance for the whole of the public services as integration is becoming increasingly important due to greater responsibility being devolved from central Government. However, for such an initiative to be successful, focusing on integration within organisations is not sufficient as real progress will require at least co-ordination if not integration of the various external performance management, assurance, audit and inspection regimes overseeing the internal governance arrangements.

Within today's society there is also an increasing emphasis on ethics including sustainability and corporate social responsibility. Both in the private, third and public sector ethics are now being considered as an integral part of management decision making. However, in practice, the issue of ethical decision making is not that easy and straight forward when designing and delivering services around service users' needs and within finite resources. Within the private sector it is argued[34] that the recommendations from the various governance reports do not necessarily provide effective models for ethical corporate governance. For the public services the question therefore remains as to whether adherence to the current principles of good governance will be enough to meet the challenges of tomorrow.

References

1 Audit Commission. *Corporate Governance Framework*. London: HMSO; 2005.
2 Cadbury Code. *Report of the Committee on the Financial Aspects of Corporate Governance: the code of best practice*. London: Gee Professional Publishing; 1992.
3 OECD. *Principles of Corporate Governance*. France: OECD; 2004.
4 Solomon J, Solomon A. *Corporate Governance and Accountability*. Chichester: John Wiley and Sons; 2004.
5 Hampel report. Final Report. *The Committee on Corporate Governance*. London: Gee Publishing; 1998.
6 Turnbull Report. *Internal Control: guidance for directors on the combined code*. London: Institute of Chartered Accountants in England and Wales; 1999.
7 Smith Report. *Audit Committees: a report and proposed guidance*. London: Financial Reporting Council; 2003.
8 Higgs Report. *Review of the Role and Effectiveness of Non-Executive Directors*. London: Department of Trade and Industry; 2003.
9 Financial Services Authority. *Combined Code of the Committee on Corporate Governance*. London: FSA; 2004
10 Audit Commission. *Corporate Governance: improvement and trust in local public services. Understanding Corporate Governance*. London: HMSO; 2003.
11 Audit Commission. *Governing Partnerships. Bridging the Accountability Gap*. London: HMSO; 2005.
12 Independent Commission for Good Governance in Public Services. OPM and CIPFA. London: 2004.
13 ACEVO, Charity Trustee Networks. ICSA, NCVO on behalf of the National Hub of Expertise in Governance. Good Governance. *A Code for the Voluntary and Community Sector*. London: NCVO; 2005.
14 Committee on Standards in Public Life. Principles of Conduct. London: HMSO;1996.
15 Scrivens E. *Quality, Risk and Control in Health Care*. Oxford: Open University Press; 2005.
16 Department of Health. *A First Class Service – quality in the new NHS*. London: HMSO;1998.
17 Scally G, Donaldson L. Clinical Governance and the drive for quality improvement in the new England. *BMJ* 1998; **317**: 61–5.
18 Department of Health. *The New NHS Modern and Dependable*. London: HMSO; 1997.
19 Department of Health. *The NHS Plan; a plan for investment, a plan for reform*. London: HMSO; 2000.
20 Department of Health. *Clinical Governance: in the New NHS*. London: HMSO; 1999.
21 Squires A. From Clinical Governance to Integrated Governance. In: Jones R, Jenkins F, editors. *Managing and Leading in the Allied Health Professions*. Oxford: Radcliffe Publishing; 2006.
22 Department of Health. HSC (98)/074.

23 www.healthcarecommission.org.uk.
24 Department of Health. *Standards for Better Health*. London: HMSO; 2004.
25 Department of Health. *Research Governance Framework for Health and Social Care*. London: HMSO; 2005.
26 Skelcher C, Mathur N, Smith M. The Public Governance of Collaborative Spaces: discourse, design and democracy. *Public Adm.* 2005; **83**(3): 573–96.
27 Health and Social Care. *Joint Guidance on governance arrangements for partnerships under the Health Act Section 31*. Advisory Note 2: Corporate governance and integrated working. London: HMSO; 2000.
28 www.integratedcarenetwork.gov.uk.
29 Audit Commission. *A fruitful partnership: effective partnership working*. London: HMSO; 1998.
30 Audit Commission Bulletin. *Developing Productive Partnerships*. London: HMSO; 2002.
31 Huczynski A, Buchanan D. *Organizational Behaviour*. Harlow: Prentice Hall; 2001.
32 Moore R. Integrated Governance Workshop. *Non-Exec Bulletin*. 2004; **5**: 6–7.
33 Department of Health. *Integrated Governance Handbook*. London: HMSO; 2006.
34 Wearing R. *Cases in Corporate Governance*. London: Sage Publications; 2005.

Annexe: corporate governance – questions and answers

Robert Jones and Fiona Jenkins

An essential element of corporate governance is communication of the organisation's values, standards and responsibilities to staff. Organisations must have rules, regulations and procedures in place relating to the conduct of business and financial procedures.

We have set out a series of questions, with answers that exemplify some key points which readers may find helpful to further understand this topic.

Q 1:   What is the quorum of a Trust Board for voting members?
A: Generally one third.

Q 2:   How often are Board members asked to update their declaration of interest?
A: At every meeting – usually monthly.

Q 3:   Whose responsibility is it, under standing orders, to disclose a relationship with other employees of the Trust, when applying for a job?
A: The applicant.

Q 4: Who is not permitted to open formal tenders?
A: The manager of the department to which the tender relates.

Q 5: You are offered a personal financial gift from a grateful patient, is it permissible to accept it?
A: No.
    Q: Should you declare the offer?
    A: Yes, you must.

Q 6: You are offered a personal financial gift by a company that supplies consumables to your department, is it permissible to accept it?
A: No.
    Q: Should you declare the offer?
    A: Yes.
    Q: Should you continue to do business with the company?
    A: There is no reason why you shouldn't, as long as you have declared the incident.

Q 7: In awarding contracts, what is the prime criterion to be applied when making the decision?
A: Financial and service merit.

Q 8: Which of these powers are reserved to the Board?
Approve annual budget ✔
Approve compensation payments ✗

Q 9: To whom is authority delegated to open bank accounts for the organisation?
A: Finance director only.

Q 10: Who is charged with monitoring compliance with Standing Orders and Standing Financial Instructions (SFIs)?
A: Trust Audit Committee.

Q 11: Who must agree proposals for use of private finance to fund a capital scheme, according to SFIs?
A: The Trust Board.

Q 12: According to SFIs, who has responsibility for the security of Trust property?
A: All employees.

Q 13: Who is responsible for the procedures and systems used to regulate stores?
A: The finance director.

Q 14: Who, according to counter fraud policies, has responsibility for the investigation of allegations of fraud?
A: The local counter fraud specialist.

Q 15: If an employee suspects a fraud, what should they do?
A: Make an immediate note of their concerns. Feed their suspicion up the management line promptly.

Q 16: If suspicion of fraud has been reported to you as the manager, what must you do?
A: Note the details of the concerns. Feed your suspicions up the management line promptly.

Q 17: When can 'hospitality' be accepted?
A: Where there is no possibility of inducement. It must be declared.
Trivial gifts such as calendars, stationery and mugs may be accepted.

Q 18: Hospitality which is offered or accepted must be declared and recorded in the Trust's hospitality register, which is kept by whom?
A: Generally the secretary to the Trust Board.
> **Q**: Hospitality which is offered or accepted must be declared, but who monitors and reviews such declarations?
> **A**: The finance director.

Q 19: Senior employees in the Trust are required to make annual declarations of their personal interests or those of close relatives. Typically who is responsible for reviewing these declarations?
A: The director of corporate services or similar director level post

Acknowledgement

East Sussex Hospitals NHS Trust. Standing Orders, SFIs and Corporate Governance Guidance; 2007.

Chapter 9
═══════════════════════════════════════

Organisational behaviour: understanding people in healthcare organisations

Sharon Mickan and Rosalie A Boyce

Introduction

One of the major reasons for looking at organisational behaviour theories is to better understand and manage people, change and teams. In order to understand a particular issue within any organisation it may be useful to view it from more than one perspective. The provision of health services must be considered in the context of healthcare organisations. Interactions between practitioners and patients occur in an organisational and social context and within a system of infrastructure. These contextual differences exist in a unique space and time within and across nations. The provision of care for any specific diagnostic group of patients is influenced by where, when and with whom it is happening. It will also depend on the availability of technical and financial resources; for example healthcare practices vary according to whether the patient was hospitalised in the 1960s or at the present time. Current practices in developing countries will differ greatly from the nature of services available in specialist clinics in industrialised metropolitan centres. Healthcare also varies according to whether the patient interacts with a single practitioner or an interdisciplinary team.

While there may be consistencies in many of the interactions between patient and professionals, and whilst there may be standardisation of practice around a pathway of care for specific diagnostic conditions, the way that healthcare is organised and delivered can be dramatically different at the end point – the service user. A suite of financial methodologies such as case mix and output-based funding are all designed to use financial drivers to reduce variations in care across settings.[1] These variations in the experience of healthcare are largely driven by the differences in the internal organisation of healthcare agencies and the subsequent impact on human behaviour.[2,3] Organisations have become exemplars for the study of occupations and organisational behaviour.[4]

> ... we would argue that the modern healthcare system is the most exciting setting in which to study work and organisations. It is a dynamic, technologically-rich environment, which incorporates interfaces between the public, private and voluntary sectors and entails a complex division of labour comprising professions, occupations, unwaged caregivers, managers and technicians. As such, it provides a natural laboratory for the exploration

of many classic sociological problems and the identification of new lines of analysis.[4]

Organisational behaviour is a way of understanding how people deal with being part of organisations. It represents a systematic approach to managing and organising people – through understanding better how they work in organisations, both as individuals and in small and large groups – managers can improve both the conditions of work and the organisations in which they work.[5] Theories that underpin organisational behaviour derive from many disciplines including sociology, organisational theory and psychology and they have changed and developed over time as analytical techniques have evolved.[6]

In this chapter the nature of health organisations is examined and the historical development of organisational behaviour theories is outlined. The text also summarises a selection of theoretical approaches and demonstrates that in most settings more than one approach guides practice. While most research in healthcare has focused on clinical issues, there is also a burgeoning interest in organisational behaviour research. A selection of research results is presented to support and exemplify these theories. Using the knowledge of a range of independent theories, readers will be able to assess the inherent conflicts within every organisation. This framework is a useful way to begin to analyse healthcare organisations. Following the theoretical sections of the chapter we apply this knowledge to recent organisational restructuring within the AHPs. This highlights the unique environmental contexts in which AHP managers work. The chapter concludes with recommendations to assist managers to work with their staff in organisational change reforms and the establishment of team based models of service provision.

Healthcare organisations

Healthcare organisations, like some other organisations, are challenged to define and measure output, where the nature of work is highly variable, complex, exacting, reactive, urgent and non-deferrable. They require a complex organisational milieu, to co-ordinate the highly specialised and differentiated professionals, who, because of the increasing complexity of healthcare, are required to work interdependently with each other.[5] Further, healthcare organisations exist in highly political environments where there is increasing competition for scarce resources.[7] Patterns of professional political power also influence the education and socialisation processes of many disciplines. Professionals' expertise and reputation influences their authority and expectation of greater autonomy and control in organisational settings. As a result, greater emphasis is placed on clinical issues, often at the expense of managerial efficiency.[8]

There has also been significant change in the composition of the healthcare workforce. At the beginning of the 20th century, physicians accounted for approximately 1:3 healthcare workers. However, by the early 1980s, the ratio had fallen to about 1:16. There has been a dramatic increase in the number and type of non-physician clinicians, which include AHP and nursing staff.[9] These non-physician clinicians have created new roles for themselves in the health workforce by providing holistic care for the chronically ill, frail elderly persons, and family caregivers. These changes have boosted inter-disciplinary collaboration and there has been a decline in the proportion of patients treated exclusively by any one clinician. In addition, there is pressure to move clinical services out of hospitals into Primary Care and to create larger organisations through mergers[10] that require more management and to consolidate services into integrated care. There have been rising public expectations of the benefits of medical care, health promotion, and disease prevention. The burden of illness has shifted from acute to chronic conditions, older patients and more technologically complex care.[11]

Although a significant amount of healthcare depends on predictable production processes as delineated in evidence-based practice and clinical guidelines, the organisation and management of healthcare cannot be interpreted similarly. Managers must look to alternative theories of management to better understand their organisations and to determine their most potent roles within them. Component areas of an organisation often adopt different theoretical approaches in order to manage the complexity of health services. Critical evaluation of these theoretical perspectives contributes to the ability to understand and enlighten current practice.

Historical development of organisational behavioural theories

Theories of scientific management and the study of bureaucracy were developed in the early 20th century. The science of management was an attempt to systematically analyse human behaviour at work. Scientific management, taken to its extreme, conceptualised people as components in an organisational machine. Work tasks were broken down into their smallest component units and analysed to promote efficiency and prevent wastage or duplication. The interaction between individuals, their social and physical environment and the task itself were all analysed to streamline and reduce unnecessary human variability. Organisations were largely predictable and they could best be understood by breaking them down into their component parts.[12] As a consequence of this approach, new levels of middle managers were required to plan and manage these operations. In healthcare environments this theory supports the detailed analysis of component administrative and clinical processes in order to streamline and improve productivity in specific areas, for example patient booking systems and the organisation of day surgeries. Through detailed analysis of the component processes, efficient pathways can be developed, implemented and evaluated. This approach is commonly used for process improvement or quality activities and is a useful strategy for healthcare managers. However, alone it is insufficient to maintain a service or to ensure sustained change.

In contrast, the study of bureaucracy sought to define whole organisations through their levels of internal authority. Hierarchies have clearly established lines of responsibility and authority, where individuals are allocated their positions according to their technical competence. A sense of stability and predictability is generated through careful management and adherence to procedures. Individuals' power, status and decision making ability are determined by their position in the hierarchy.[5] Traditionally, healthcare organisations have been bureaucratically arranged, with the medical profession having had a dominant role. Doctors have used a range of informal and formalised peer group systems to define and rank nursing and AHP positions in the hierarchy.[8] However, more recently, a range of parallel professional multi-layered hierarchies have challenged healthcare systems, structures and processes, resulting in varying lines of responsibility and operational procedures.[13]

Bureaucratic and scientific theories have strongly influenced both the practice of medicine and the leadership and management of organisations. However, these theories on their own are most helpful when there is a high level of predictability about the task, for example, cardiac resuscitation and hip replacement surgery.[12] These theories are also helpful when there is agreement from those working together about what is required, how it will happen and what can be expected.[14]

With the increasing prevalence of the broad field of psychology in the 1930s, comparatively mechanistic views were complemented by a more humanistic approach, which focused on the behaviour of people in work groups. Human relations/resource theory highlights the way in which individual levels of motivation, satisfaction, creativity and productivity can be enhanced when there are appropriate and supportive structures and management processes. Managers are encouraged to develop good communication and collaboration skills to maximise individuals' motivation and participation, particularly in solving localised organisation problems. Performance management systems are commonly used to motivate and manage employees, although internal bureaucracies can negatively influence their implementation. These strategies have become increasingly common in healthcare organisations particularly in areas where there is a focus on promoting teamwork. Currently, many healthcare organisations actively empower and motivate individuals to provide quality patient care through supporting continuing personal development and professional education and integrating evidence-based practice through research.

Literature analysis suggests that there are three human resource practices positively associated with organisational performance:

1 appraisal
2 training
3 teamworking.[15]

Extensive appraisal systems that focus on improving goal setting and feedback processes help employees direct, correct and improve their performance. Training in technical, clinical and leadership skills has been shown to improve individual and organisational performance.[16] Working in teams has been linked to better quality patient care in primary health and community mental healthcare teams. Furthermore, team working enables clearer role definition, more effective inter-disciplinary interaction, higher levels of job satisfaction and better mental health for team members.[17] These benefits have been confirmed by comparison with patient mortality data in a study of 61 acute hospitals in England. It is possible to influence hospital performance significantly by implementing extensive appraisal and training systems and encouraging staff to work in teams.[15]

During the 1960s systems theory developed as a way of describing the complex interdependence of relationships within organisations. Generally, a system comprises regularly interacting or interrelating parts, which together form a new whole. Often, the whole is greater than, and different from, its constituent parts. A systems view of organisations transcends and integrates individual perspectives/disciplines, and focuses on the internal processes, rather than the elements of the system. From an analysis of these dynamic interrelationships new properties of the system emerge. Importantly, 'open systems' emphasise the links between organisations and their external environments, thereby highlighting the need for organisations to be adaptable and innovative.[13] Systems theory is also important in promoting learning and adaptation. As organisations learn about their environments, they can adapt themselves to the environment and ensure their longevity.[7] Many new organisational behavioural theories have emerged since this time to emphasise certain components of the environment.[18] Generally, these theories interpret different aspects of the environment.

Resource dependence theory states that organisations need to adapt to both political and financial environments. Internal power and influence is related to access to key external resources. Organisations that become dependent on their environment for crucial resources will experience greater uncertainty. They must therefore reduce dependence on the external environment as much as possible by controlling resources. Organisations can conversely increase the dependence of agents in their environment on their own unique and distinctive services and products.[7] Depending on the environmental levels of uncertainty, organisations may compete to increase their influence and control of scarce resources or they might join with other organisations to pool resources. Complex and unstable environments in healthcare where there are changing resources have resulted in the emergence of a range of relationships between organisations, from informal information sharing to fully operational mergers.[19] While hospitals have longstanding interactions with both the politics and economics of government, there has been a strong move to make these interactions more transparent and ultimately accountable.

An alternative open systems theory 'institutional theory', explains that organisations succeed and prosper through obtaining a good 'fit' between the organisation and its external environment.[20] Organisations gain legitimacy by adapting to and adopting work procedures that are well accepted in their environments, and therefore they obtain the resources they need for their survival.[7] Successful organisations also adopt the norms, rules and values of key external stakeholders to fit better into their environments and increase their prospects of survival.[21] Health services organisations have relatively fixed ideas about behaviours and standards that should operate. As a consequence there are also many widely held or rationalised beliefs that certain behaviours are important. Sometimes there is conflict in prioritising these. Increasingly, healthcare organisations are being required to communicate with and meet the needs of these diverse stakeholder groups.

Since the 1980s relational concepts of organisations have become increasingly popular, due to the recognition of the interdependence of processes within and beyond organisations.[18] For example, the perspective of strategic management emphasises the importance of organisations managing their internal and external environments in a positive manner. Strategic management incorporates a logical process of thinking, analysis, planning and evaluation, which takes organisations from defining their purpose to planning how they will achieve their chosen objectives. Careful definition and monitoring of goal achievement enables progress towards the organisation's desired outcomes.[22] Therefore, information systems are vital in improving managers' abilities to better predict and plan for desired outcomes. The 'Balanced Scorecard' is an implementation and monitoring tool where an organisation's strategy becomes the key for focusing and aligning staff. The intangible internal knowledge, capabilities and relationships between staff are captured through a limited set of key performance indicators. Regular measurement and management of these indicators enables organisations to plan for and achieve significant success.[23]

During the last few decades, chaos, quantum and complexity theories have provided alternative explanations of organisational change to accommodate some of the limitations of rational analysis and provide insights into the management of healthcare systems.[24,25] Complex adaptive systems are characterised by a number of elements interacting locally in a fluid, flexible and non-linear manner. Each system influences and is influenced by other systems, and not necessarily in a linear way. Small changes may have large effects or vice versa and therefore detailed planning and prediction is not always possible. Order and rules evolve through a balance between competition and co-operation without the need for hierarchical systems of control. Systems are often unpredictable and move towards self-organisation, such that mutually beneficial relationships grow and develop and appropriate structures emerge. Systems may adapt to change and then contribute to subsequent change.

Kernick[12] suggested that there are some counter-intuitive patterns within complexity theory. He suggests that every organisation has a 'shadow organisation' which sets the rules of engagement, beyond and sometimes unrelated to the legitimate hierarchies, rules and communication patterns. This might explain why there are some people in every organisation who have more or less power than their hierarchical position would suggest. Every organisation has a unique history which influences the way it develops and the way decisions are made. Therefore, two similar organisations may have very different cultures due to their divergent histories.[26] Complex systems typically have poorly defined boundaries where membership can change and individuals may be members of more than one system or set of relationships – this is common in AHPs where individual professionals often belong to both professional and clinical systems. These systems also incorporate creativity and other emergent phenomena.[14]

Kernick[12] further suggested that complexity theory is most beneficial when there is limited predictability in the environment. For example, when there is uncertainty how outputs can be measured and how inputs are converted to outputs. In these situations complexity theory can facilitate an understanding of what creates behaviours and patterns of order, it describes how patterns evolve and suggest insights about how to promote desirable change and limit undesirable effects. It moves the emphasis of analysis away from prediction and control to identifying relationships and looking for the source of the inherent patterns of order and behaviour in these relationships. It is particularly helpful in facilitating understanding of the relationships between components of the system. For example, complexity based organisational thinking suggests that improved patient care could be established by looking at the whole health system, across funding and management boundaries. Rather than an acute hospital setting unrealistic targets for emergency care that the ambulance services cannot meet, a more realistic plan, incorporating minimum specifications, could be generated through communication with both services.[14]

At the same time, a range of contingency approaches have become popular to better understand the contingency or unexplained influences between management style, organisational structure and environmental aspects – there may not be 'one best way' for organisation, management and leadership. Organisations that 'fit' contextual features such as size, technology and structure of their environment are more likely to perform well and therefore survive longer.[7]

Situational leadership theories propose that specific leadership styles are better in different situations and therefore, leaders must be flexible enough to adapt their styles to the situations they find themselves in. An effective leader is one who can quickly adapt leadership styles as the situations change.[27] The Aston School emphasises the need to measure and explain the relationships between an organisation's structure and a range of contextual variables. They found that common denominators exist across these structural variations and can be applied to a wide range of organisations concluding that people and their performance are crucial for an organisation's success.[28]

Organisational boundaries are often blurred and may change in response to their environments. Several approaches from organisational behaviour theory can enhance understanding of organisations, their environment and the behaviour of the staff. NHS management restructuring has seen the emergence of a horizontal method of internal organisation – 'flat structures' – in which strategies include management through networks, partnership working and process redesign.[29]

Impact on healthcare managers

It may be helpful for AHP managers to be aware of some theoretical approaches. For example, an understanding of 'scientific management principles' could influence thinking when designing a new service. Human resource theories suggest that participation in decision making leads to high levels of employee satisfaction, which in turn leads to increased productivity. Effective participation takes place when employees have the competence and motivation to contribute, and are given an opportunity to do so.[28] However, it may also be useful to consider strategic management and contingency theories for example.

It may also be useful for AHP managers to be aware of institutional theories. Managers need to keep themselves informed about management and organisational trends in and beyond healthcare organisations. While it is not possible to ascertain which management and organisational trends will prosper and last the test of time, managers need to be able to respond constructively to new strategies. Managers can often identify new growth and development opportunities such as developing unique services and added value programmes.

Conforming to new institutional rules and procedures can be detrimental to professional practice.[30] AHP managers need to have the ability to 'hold their own' in changing circumstances and contribute to actively shape new priorities, structures and processes. Managers need to be actively involved in executive level decision making processes where possible. It is also vital that the needs of patients are upheld in all circumstances particularly in aspects of conflicting priorities. Furthermore managers may be able to reduce their dependence on the traditional income streams to some extent and diversify their funding, through exploiting these opportunities.[31] Healthcare systems experience an inherent tension between the need for predictability, order and efficiency of their internal systems, and the need to be responsive, flexible and strategic with respect to their external environments. In practice, managers must develop objectives, choose strategies and implement structures that are consistent with both their external environments and internal capabilities.

It is also important that managers look to their environment to contribute to their organisation's performance. Organisations need to be able to respond rapidly to changing events and needs in the environment. However, individual staff may be vulnerable, stressed and have less job stability or security.[32] In contrast, stable organisations can develop clear hierarchies of roles and authority, formal organisational and communication structures and ultimately provide security and stability for staff.[7] Traditionally, healthcare organisations in the developed world have functioned within stable environments. However, this stability is no longer a certainty and there is a need for many healthcare organisations to adapt to increasingly turbulent situations. As healthcare costs rise and technology develops and increases, governments are paying increasingly large proportions of their gross national product for healthcare. Therefore, there is increasing competition for limited resources and organisations' needs and expectations are constantly being re-evaluated. Arguably bureaucracies will progressively be replaced by more flexible and organic organisational structures that can adapt quickly to rapidly changing environments.[32] However, such a transformation will not proceed rapidly.

At the same time, managers need to be more creative and innovative, particularly in the face of competing stakeholder expectations. They cannot ignore the claims of complexity theories and situational management and must adapt their behaviour to different circumstances. Managers need to be able to work across a spectrum of environments. They should aim to maintain stability in their services as much as possible and survive the challenging aspects of enforced change.[7] With the increasing complexity in healthcare provision there has been growth in the specialisation and fragmentation of care. As practitioners become more specialised, there are increasing costs and a greater number of communication and co-ordination strategies required which add to the overall complexity. There are likely to be new ways of organising in the future. It may be professional groups or administrative managers that lead these changes. However, there will need to be significant and well informed dialogue between all parties.

A comprehensive theoretical framework

Some research studies suggest that changing organisational culture is a way to improve the quality, efficiency, patient focus and performance of healthcare organisations.[2] However, the quality of research is hindered by the inherent difficulties in defining and measuring these complex constructs. It is also not clear whether organisational culture or performance is the pre-cursor. Most importantly, it is imperative to recognise that there is a broad heterogeneity of healthcare organisations and that no one theoretical approach or description can describe all or even most organisations. Whilst the earlier discussion about a variety of theories is useful, it benefits from consolidation into a more comprehensive theoretical framework.

Organisational behavioural theorists recognise that there is inherent tension and competition between many theories. While it is important to consider these differences, it can be difficult to resolve the many intrinsic dichotomies. However, an alternative framework has been developed to recognise the specific situations that promote effectiveness within organisations. A competing values framework enables recognition of two sets of competing demands.[33] On the one hand, there is tension between focusing on 'people versus the organisation' as a whole. On the other hand there are competing demands for structure and stability, compared to flexibility and responsiveness.[33,34,35] The juxtaposition of these two dimensions results in four organisational cultural orientations as shown in Table 9.1.

- Group.
- Open.
- Rational.
- Hierarchical.

While these cultures are described as 'ideal' types, they are likely to be reflected to varying degrees in different organisations. Often, organisations reflect a combination of each cultural type with one or two cultures being more dominant than others. Conversely, each culture emphasises different organisational activities and therefore different criteria of effectiveness. It is beneficial for managers to consider which type best reflects their organisation, to identify which are the dominant approaches.

1 Group culture is derived from a high degree of flexibility and focus on people. It emphasises teamwork, cohesiveness and participation. This culture promotes commitment and morale, mentoring and rewarding people for being team players. Management strategies may include creating special clinical teams to focus on particular issues and developing educational programmes.
2 Open culture represents a high focus on flexibility and the organisation. It is characterised by the promotion of innovation, risk taking and growth. Entrepreneurial and risk taking leaders are supported and people are rewarded for taking and sharing risk. Pilot programmes may be developed and encouraged. Opinion leaders may be sought out and encouraged to lead change initiatives.
3 Rational culture is derived from a focus on control and on the organisation. It emphasises the achievement of objectives through gaining competitive advantage. People are rewarded for acquiring the resources to achieve organisational goals. Clinical protocols and guidelines may be frequently used. Expert advice from, for example, professional bodies is considered important.
4 Hierarchical culture represents a focus on control and people. Emphasising stability, rules and regulations. People are rewarded for adhering to policies and leaders are supported for emphasising order and achieving operational predictability. Often strategies of performance management and peer review are widely used. Performance feedback is important both for information and comparative evaluation.[36]

Each of these cultural types aids understanding of healthcare organisations. On their own, each culture identifies key organisational goals, values, leadership styles and strategic emphases. Each culture has a tendency to improve performance on aspects that are particularly valued in that culture. For example,[37] hospitals with dominant group cultures performed significantly above average on measures of employee loyalty and commitment. Hospitals with dominant open cultures performed better on measures of external stakeholder satisfaction and

Table 9.1 Competing values framework.

	Flexibility focus	
Group Culture **Staff climate:** cohesiveness, participation, teamwork, sense of belonging **Leadership styles:** mentor, facilitator **Values:** loyalty, tradition, cohesion **Strategic emphases:** human resource development, commitment, staff morale		*Open Culture* **Staff climate:** creative, entrepreneurial, adaptable, dynamic **Leadership styles:** entrepreneur, innovator, risk-taker **Values:** entrepreneurship, flexibility, risk, readiness **Strategic emphases:** innovation, growth
People focus		Organisation focus
Hierarchy Culture **Staff climate:** order, rules, regulations, uniformity, efficiency, clear expectations, information management, communication **Leadership styles:** coordinator, organiser, administrator **Values:** adherence to policies and procedures **Strategic emphases:** stability, predictability, smooth operations		*Rational Culture* **Staff climate:** competitive, goal setting and achievement, planning **Leadership styles:** decisive, focus on production and achievement, expert **Values:** clear goals, production, competition **Strategic emphases:** predictable, productive, competitive advantage, market superiority
	Control focus	

those with dominant hierarchical cultures were more internally consistent. Managers can use this to better understand their organisation. While a hierarchical culture emphasises stability and rules it aims to maintain the 'current order'. Change is likely to be interpreted as threatening and therefore it can be predicted that hierarchical organisations are unlikely to be initiators of change. However, these organisations can be influenced towards incremental structural change that focuses on people within the structures.

It is likely that each organisation has one or two dominant cultures at any one time. Hospital management teams in the UK[37] were more frequently group and hierarchical cultures, whereas American hospital teams were more likely to be rational and open cultures. Canadian teams were more often group and rational cultures. In another study,[35] it was found that hospitals which scored high on adaptability, flexibility and growth reported greater involvement in quality improvement and implementation activities. Therefore, critical analysis of healthcare organisations in terms of this theoretical framework will identify which cultural and performance issues are likely to be most valued and show improvement. The earlier theoretical models may also shed more light on particular issues within an organisation.

It may be helpful for managers to map out their environments, so that they are aware of strengths, weaknesses, opportunities and threats. Efforts need to be balanced as much as possible between all these quadrants and between internal and external environments. It is also important to manage resource dependencies to ensure a steady flow of resources, mindful that when one income stream is reduced, opportunities for alternatives can be developed.

Clinical governance and human resource management strategies improves the quality of patient care through both individual and organisational initiatives.[38] As the volume of activity increases within health related groups benefits and performance efficiencies are observed as staff become more practised in managing and caring for a particular patient group. Contingency theory suggests that some managerial approaches would work for some groups of patients and types of services and not for others. NHS Trusts also differ in the extent to which departments such as finance and human resources staff are devolved from professional departments into wider management teams. The extent to which medical staff are involved in management is also a distinguishing feature of some NHS Trusts, which might have a bearing on power sharing and levels of responsibility.

AHP structures

Organisational behaviour impacts on the development of management structures throughout the services including AHPs.

Management arrangements for AHPs are not uniform across the NHS. In some places a single head of service manages each of the professions as individual entities. In others they are managed in a variety of different groupings, for example in directorate structures or in combined AHP groups, either within one trust or across several trusts. The management role is sometimes divided between management and professional functions. Theses roles are sometimes separated and may be undertaken by different individuals not necessarily from the same professional backgrounds.[39]

> **Editors' note**
>
> AHP organisational and management structures in the UK and Australia are explored, analysed and discussed in detail in Chapters 1–6 of *Managing and Leading in the Allied Health Professions*, the first book in this series 'Allied Health Professions – Essential Guides'.[40]

Practical perspectives

Most managers begin their analysis of organisational behaviour at the level in which they are working. However, it is advisable to analyse the situation from both the level above and the level below, to better understand the whole situation.[41] Often clinicians from all disciplines are used to reducing problems to their component parts to better understand them. Increasingly, in unpredictable environments this alone is not sufficient. Therefore, it is important to look at the situation from a higher level. By comparing all three perspectives there will be an enriched understanding of what is really going on. Often reasons emerge that may have escaped notice in the analysis of only one or two levels. Patterns may be determined at higher levels, such as within the dynamics or relationships of an organisational culture or even at the level of composition of the organisation.[26] From a contingency theory perspective it is necessary to examine the patterns of common or rhythmic qualities. This assists in identifying a range of improvement strategies.

The transition to managing people

One of the ways in which organisational culture and 'climate' affect employee behaviour is through its influence on people management.[28] It is argued that all healthcare managers are under increasing pressure from social, economic and political factors, within a broad context of reform. In addition to providing high quality clinical services, clinical managers must also adopt a strong managerial perspective to improve performance in line with key organisational outcomes. At times it appears that professional autonomy is in conflict with managerial objectives. These dual roles lead to tension between familiar professional values of clinical autonomy on the one hand and managerial demands for improved efficiency and cost control on the other. It is therefore an enduring challenge for managers to resolve the potential for conflict between these two conflicting notions of management and professional independence.

Clinical staff need management education, knowledge, skills training and socialisation into management roles. Too often in healthcare organisations there is limited management education and training, combined with a lack of clear role expectations. The way in which managers with clinical backgrounds approach their management roles is often influenced by previous role models, existing role conflicts and the extent to which clinicians choose to become managers.[30]

To make the transition from clinician to manager, changes in behaviour may be required. Positive aspects of working in combined clinical and managerial environments need to be realised. There are likely to be opportunities for AHP managers to establish relationships between different healthcare professionals and with administrative managers. There may also be opportunities to influence the ways that professionals practice and use resources. Creative problem solving and analysis may generate alternative ways of organising clinical work. AHP managers can advocate for more flexible skill mixes to reflect the organisation's clinical patterns and priorities.[32] In addition, they may have good opportunities to be entrepreneurial.[31] Through understanding their own organisation's culture and key environmental issues, managers can develop new services, look for alternative means of funding services and better meet otherwise unmet patient need. It can be valuable for managers to review their organisation according to one or more theoretical perspective to identify what is important and valuable for current and future service provision.

Perspectives on managing people

Editors' note

Concepts of leadership are discussed in detail by Christina Pond in Chapter 7 Leadership in the Allied Health Professions *of Managing and Leading in the Allied Health Professions*, the first book in the Allied Health Professions – Essential Guides series.[40]

It is important to consider the concepts of leadership and education from an organisational behaviour perspective. Leadership is included only briefly here. Contingency theories suggest that leadership style needs to change to reflect different situations. There are broad and common themes about leadership in healthcare organisations which suggest that individual leaders can have a significant effect on the organisation's performance. A focus on people management is considered important. Leaders that focus on performance management and developing trust and respect achieve better performance.[28] In contrast, poor leadership has been shown to reduce job satisfaction, organisational commitment and contribute to poor team working, psychological distress and ultimately less effective patient care.[17]

Strategies to be considered in effective leadership include:[28]

- promoting confident and optimistic attitudes to increase the enthusiasm of co-workers
- developing individual's skills
- promoting mutual appreciation for each other
- facilitating the management of conflict
- building trust within and across teams
- creating alignment around achieving the 'best' organisational outcomes.

AHP managers must identify education and training needs with their staff which should be identified through comprehensive appraisal and performance review systems. Policies and practices which include both profession specific skills training and clinical/leadership skills development must be put in place. An appreciation of organisational behaviour theory on a macro scale will enhance the manager's own behaviour in terms of managing and developing their services within the organisation as a whole and forms a useful background in the management of individuals and teams within their services.

Perspectives on change

Managers have a crucial role in facilitating their staff and colleagues through change situations. However, it is a useful exercise for clinicians who become managers to reflect on their motivation for undertaking these roles. While some clinicians choose management as a career there are also some who move into management reluctantly others who might be 'coerced' into management.[30]

Many employees have a positive attitude towards change when they can have some influence over its direction. Management support, meaningful participation and good communication are all required to enact organisational change. Employees need to be engaged in the change management process – see Chapter 2 in this book.

Different management and leadership styles influence how people experience change processes. Leaders who adopt predominantly 'democratic' styles tend to improve the morale and social aspects of work, often at the expense of productivity. In contrast, 'autocratic' leaders may achieve more productivity at the expense of individual motivation and group solidarity.[42]

Often the slow spread of a change initiative is linked to a group of people labelled 'resistors to change'. Complexity theory suggests that these people might prefer the status quo. However, they may not be actively resisting but rather focused on achieving something else. Therefore, the change leader's challenge is to better understand the motivation of individuals within the team. Leaders may initiate change processes in terms of their own motivators and fail to recognise the tensions which arise from other people's perspectives and from within the situation. Leadership inspired by complexity theory recognises that changes occur naturally and for various reasons. Therefore, the leader's role is to create systems to disseminate information about best practices and allow others to adopt these practices in ways that are meaningful to them.[14]

Perspectives on teamwork

Teams are a feature of most organisations. Therefore, the management of teams, and their processes, is a significant aspect of organisational behaviour. Teams are social groups performing tasks that contribute to the organisation's goals. Team members depend on each other to achieve their tasks. They have achievable performance goals for which they are held collectively responsible. Team membership is usually recognised by the team members themselves and also by those outside the team. Frequently AHPs belong to more than one team, for example the professional group and one or more clinical and management teams. The competing interests arising for membership of multiple teams may cause tensions and stress.[43]

AHP managers must promote effective team working and ensure, where possible, that there are clear definitions of individual and team roles. It is an increasing challenge to distinguish between core discipline specific skills and roles and shared multi-professional skills. In some areas of work, there may be specific functions where one or more disciplines could perform certain tasks.

In a study of more than 500 teams in the NHS, it was shown that teams with clear objectives, high levels of participation and task orientation, support for innovation, and time available for review were more effective in delivering patient care.[17] 'Innovative' teams demonstrated high levels of professional diversity and a variety of work functions. Their team 'climate' was characterised by shared vision, participative decision making, constructive management of conflict, tolerance of minority dissent, internal trust and safety and support for innovation. These teams also took time to review their performance and made changes accordingly. Team members were to some extent 'buffered' from the negative effects of adverse organisational 'climate' and conflict and were more likely to stay working in effective teams.

The development of teams requires high level organisational support. Systems need to be geared towards managing teams as well as individuals, in relation to communication, education, people management and rewards. Ideally power, control responsibility and accountability should be devolved to the level of teams. However this can be difficult to achieve in healthcare organisations.

Conclusion

It is helpful to consider all aspects of an organisation's environment. Using organisational behaviour theories and frameworks to better understand and analyse what is important for a particular organisation taking into account both internal and external environments and factors. Having an awareness of theories such as scientific, bureaucratic and human resource theories can help to facilitate managerial practice together with evaluating the level of strategic management including the key visions, directions and plans for the organisation. Where there is greater complexity and variability look for recurring patterns across different levels of the organisation and consider contingencies. The nature of AHP management, leadership and clinical service provision continues to evolve in line with the many changes within and outside the NHS, thoughtfully applied organisational behaviour perspectives will contribute to the knowledge base and help managers and leaders to better undertake their roles.

References

1 Courtney M, Briggs D. *Healthcare Financial Management*. Marrickville, Australia: Elsevier Mosby; 2004.
2 Elliott RF, Scott A, Skåtun D, *et al*. The impact of local labour market factors on the organisation and delivery of health services. London: NHS Service Delivery and Organisation R&D Program; 2003.
3 Kinston W. Hospital organisation and structure and its effect on inter-professional behaviour and the delivery of care. *Soc Sci Med.* 1983; **17**(16): 1159–70.
4 Allen D, Pilnick A. Making connections: healthcare as a case study in the social organisation of work. *Sociol Health Ill.* 2005; **27**(6): 683–700.
5 Anderson R, McDaniel R. Managing Healthcare organizations: where professionalism meets complexity science. *Healthcare Manage Rev.* 2000; **25**(1): 83–92.
6 Flood A, Fennell M. Through the lenses of organizational sociology: the role of organizational theory and research in conceptualizing and examining our healthcare system. *J Health Soc Behav.* 1995; Extra issue: 154–69.
7 Schmid H. Organization-environment relationships: theory for management practice in human service organizations. *Admin Soc Work.* 2004; **28**(1): 97–113.
8 Preston A, Badrick T. Organisational influences. In: Clinton M, Scheiwe D, editors. *Management in the Australian Healthcare Industry*. Melbourne: Longman; 1998.
9 Druss B, Marcus S, Olfson M. *et al*. Trends in care by nonphysician clinicians in the United States. *New Engl J Med.* 2003; **348**(2): 130–7.
10 Fulop N, Protopsaltis G, King A, *et al*. Changing organisations: a study of the context and processes of mergers of healthcare providers in England. *Soc Sci Med.* 2005; **60**(1): 119–30.
11 Aiken L. Achieving an interdisciplinary workforce in Healthcare. *New Engl J Med.* 2003; **348**(2): 164–6.
12 Kernick D. The demise of linearity in managing health services: a call for post normal Healthcare. *J Health Serv Res Policy.* 2002; **7**(2): 121–4.
13 Shortell S, Kaluzny A, editors. *Healthcare Management: organization design and behavior.* 5th ed. Clifton Park, NY: Delmar Pub; 2005.
14 Plsek P, Greenhalgh T. The challenge of complexity in healthcare. *Brit Med J.* 2001; **323**:625–8.
15 West M, Borrill C, Dawson J, *et al*. The link between the management of employees and patient mortality in acute hospitals. *Int J Hum Res Man.* 2002; **13**(8): 1299–310.
16 Morrow C, Jarrett M. An investigation of the effect and economic utility of corporate-wide training. *Pers Psychol* 1997; **46**: 91–119.
17 Borrill C, West M, Dawson J, *et al*. Team working and effectiveness in healthcare. *Brit J Healthcare.* 2000; **6**: 364–71.
18 Scott W. Reflections on a half-century of organizational sociology. *Ann Rev Sociol.* 2004; **30**:1–21.

19 Salancik G, Pfeffer J. Who gets power – and how they hold on to it: a strategic-contingencies model of power. *Organ Dyn.* 1977; **5**: 3–21.

20 Powell W, DiMaggio P. *The New Institutionalism in Organizational Analysis.* Chicago: University of Chicago Press; 1991.

21 Daft R, Lewin A. Can organizational studies begin to break out of the normal science straight jacket? *Organ Sci.* 1990; **1**: 1–10.

22 Biscoe G, Lewis B. Strategic thinking and business planning. In: Clinton M, Scheiwe D, editors. *Management in the Australian Healthcare Industry.* 2nd ed. Melbourne: Longman; 1998.

23 Kaplan R, Norton D. *The Strategy-Focused Organization: how balanced scorecard companies thrive in the new business environment.* Boston, MA: Harvard Business School Press; 2001.

24 Bigelow B, Arndt M. The more things change, the more they stay the same. *Healthcare Manage Rev.* 2000; **25**(1): 65–72.

25 Burnes B. Complexity theories and organizational change. *Int J Manag Rev.* 2005; **7**(2): 73–90.

26 Braithwaite J, Westbrook M. Rethinking clinical organisational structures: an attitude survey of doctors, nurses and allied health staff in clinical directorates. *J Health Services Research Policy.* 2005; **10**(1): 10–17.

27 Hersey P, Blanchard H. *Management of Organisational Behavior: utilizing human resources.* Englewood Cliffs, NJ: Prentice Hall Inc; 1993.

28 Michie S, West M. Managing people and performance: an evidence based framework applied to health service organizations. *Int J Manag Rev.* 2004; **5–6**: 91–111.

29 McNulty T, Ferlie E. Process transformation: limitations to radical organizational change within public service organizations. *Organ Studies.* 2004; **25**(8): 1389–412.

30 Forbes T, Hallier J, Kelly L. Doctors as managers: investors and reluctants in a dual role. *Health Serv Manag Res.* 2004; **17**(3): 167–176.

31 Rowe P, Boyce R, Boyle M, *et al.* A comparative analysis of entrepreneurial approaches within public healthcare organisations. *Aust J Publ Admin.* 2004; **63**(2): 16–30.

32 Hunter D. The changing roles of Healthcare personnel in health and Healthcare management. *Soc Sci Med.* 1996; **43**(5): 799–808.

33 Quinn R, Rohrbaugh J. Competing values approach to organizational effectiveness. *Public Prod Rev.* 1981; **5**(2): 122–140.

34 Scott T, Mannion R, Davies H. *et al.* Implementing culture change in healthcare: theory and practice. *Int J Qual Healthcare.* 2003; **15**(2): 111–118.

35 Gerowitz M. Do TQM interventions change management culture? Findings and implications. *Qual Manag Healthcare.* 1998; **6**(3): 1–11.

36 Wallace L, Freeman T, Latham L, *et al.* Organisational strategies for changing clinical practice: how trusts are meeting the challenges of clinical governance. *Qual Healthcare.* 2001; **10**: 76–82.

37 Gerowitz MB, Lemieux-Charles L, Heginbothan C, *et al.* Top management culture and performance in Canadian, UK and US hospitals. *Health Serv Manage Research.* 1996; **9**: 69–78.

38 West E. Management matters: the link between hospital organisation and quality of patient care. *Qual Healthcare.* 2001; **10**(1): 40–8.

39 Jones R, Jenkins F. Allied Health Professions management and organisation: what structure? In: Jones R, Jenkins F, editors. *Managing and Leading in the Allied Health Professions.* Oxford: Radcliffe Publishing; 2006.

40 Jones R, Jenkins F. *Managing and Leading in the Allied Health Professions.* Oxford: Radcliffe Publishing; 2006.

41 Hackman J. Learning more by crossing levels: Evidence from airplanes, hospitals, and orchestras. *J Organ Behav.* 2003; **24**: 905–22.

42 Cortvriend P. Change management of mergers: the impact on NHS staff and their psychological contracts. *Health Serv Manag Research.* 2004; **17**(13): 177–87.

43 Mickan S, Rodger S. Effective Healthcare Teams: a model of six characteristics developed from shared perceptions. *J Interprof Care.* 2005; **19**(4): 358–70.

Chapter 10

Managing health and safety in the workplace

Claire Sullivan

Introduction

An employer's duty to provide a safe and healthy working environment is one of the cornerstones of the contractual relationship between an organisation and its staff. Work can pose dangers to people's health, safety and welfare and the framework of health and safety law which exists in the UK aims to prevent and control such dangers, to set standards and to provide staff with some element of protection.

This chapter provides a brief overview of the UK health and safety legal framework and related matters; it has a particular focus on the likely role and responsibilities of AHP managers in managing health and safety in their own workplaces and departments.

The following pages introduce and expand on the concept of a risk-assessment based approach to all workplace health and safety matters and explore some of the most common issues and hazards facing members of the AHPs at work. The important role of safety representatives and how managers and safety representatives can work together is addressed in some detail.

It is intended that managers should be able to dip in and out of this chapter, as they face new health and safety situations and challenges in their workplaces.

Health and safety in the health services

The four key health and safety hazards in the health services which lead to the greatest number of injuries and incidences of ill-health are stress, musculoskeletal disorders, violence and slips, trips and falls.[1]

The health and social care sector has a higher than average incidence of work-related illness compared with other industries and at 2.4% this has not altered significantly in recent years. Rates for work-related infections and dermatitis in the sector are, perhaps unsurprisingly, well above average.[2]

Musculoskeletal conditions, especially spine/back disorders are an important cause of work-related illness in the sector and along with stress, depression and anxiety, exhibit some of the highest prevalence rates in any industry.

In terms of how these prevalence rates related to lost working days, these estimates are subject to some uncertainty. However, it is clear that the rate in the health sector is above the all-industry average, at an average of 1.8 days per worker per year.

As explained further on in this chapter, the law requires fatalities, certain major injuries as classified under the law, and those causing more than three consecutive days off work to be represented to the Health and Safety Executive.[3] Some of the statistics resulting from these reports are set out below:

- in the last ten years, there have been ten fatalities amongst workers in the sector
- 55% of reported major injuries in the sector are caused by slips, trips and falls
- 14% of major injuries are caused by accidents involving moving and handling
- 12% of major injuries are caused by violent attacks
- of injuries and other incidents causing more than three days off work:
  - 51% are caused by moving and handling incidents
  - 19% of these are caused by slips, trips and falls
  - 15% are caused by violent attacks.

Stress-related absences are not included in the data above.

Health and safety law in the UK

Background to the Health and Safety at Work Act

Since 1974, the central piece of health and safety law in the UK has been the Health and Safety at Work etc Act.[4] Prior to its introduction, health and safety regulations had developed in a piecemeal fashion, with a myriad of different Acts covering a range of hazards and industries and taking very differing approaches to how employers should make work safer and control risks. A Royal Commission, set up in the early 1970s to consider the future regulation of workplace health and safety – the Robens Commission – proposed radical change; the Health and Safety at Work etc Act, often referred to by the acronym 'HASAWA' introduced one broad 'umbrella' law covering all workers in every workplace, under which all more specific health and safety provisions would be enacted in the future. Some further detail of the legal standards set by HASAWA is given later in this section but its other important function was to create both the Health and Safety Commission (HSC) and the Health and Safety Executive (HSE).

The HSC, HSE and enforcing the law

The HSC is a nine-person body appointed by Government which, along with its full-time Chair, has overall responsibility for formulating health and safety law and policy. Commissioners are appointed to represent a variety of interests across industries, including those of employers and employees. The HSE is the body appointed by the Commission to implement these policy decisions and enforce the law, with day-to-day enforcement being carried out by local HSE inspectors. In 2006, a consultation document was issued on a proposal to merge the Health and Safety Commission and Executive into one body. Initial reaction from unions and many employers indicate that such a move would be widely-supported.

HSE inspectors are based in offices around the countries and have designated responsibilities for particular sectors or workplaces within their locality. As larger organisations, NHS Trusts and other healthcare establishments will usually have a named inspector allocated to them; the role of this inspector is to provide general advice and guidance and to conduct workplace inspections. Such inspections may be in response to a particular problem which has arisen in a workplace but may also be routine in nature. Routine inspections in Trusts and hospitals are planned in advance and usually involve a team of four or five inspectors visiting the Trust over several days. During this time, they will meet a range of staff, including safety representatives and managers and will look at all the policies and systems which are in place to control risk and make work safe.

If inspectors are not satisfied that all aspects of an organisation's performance comply with the expected legal standards, they may offer advice about improvements but can also take formal action to ensure such improvement takes place, by issuing 'notices'. There are two forms of legal notice – improvement and prohibition. The former sets a time by which changes must be made while the latter – for more serious breaches – prevents the particular area or activity which has been found lacking from continuing until the recommended changes have been put in place. In the most serious cases, where it is deemed that a notice would not be sufficient, the HSE can recommend a criminal prosecution of an organisation under the Health and Safety at Work Act.

Understanding what the law means

At first glance, health and safety law can seem complicated and impenetrable and managers could be forgiven for feeling no wiser after reading a document spelling out their legal duties than they did beforehand. This section addresses the need to de-mystify the relevant law; with practise it is no different from learning to understand medical terminology! Health and safety law is peppered with words and phrases which recur throughout and once you know the correct 'recipe' these are helpful rather than confusing.

Under HASAWA, all health and safety law is divided into Regulations, Approved Codes of Practice (ACOPs) and Guidance Notes.

Regulations: all of the more specific 'laws' which are enacted under the umbrella of HASAWA are in the form of regulations. While they pass through Parliament more quickly than an Act – they are implemented as Statutory Instruments – they have the full force of the law and it is legally binding for employers to comply with their requirements in full. Regulations are often reasonably brief and general.

For example, Regulation 2 of the Workplace – Health, Safety and Welfare – Regulations 1992 states:

Suitable and sufficient sanitary conveniences shall be provided at readily accessible places.

ACOPs: regulations are often accompanied by an ACOP, which gives more detail on *how* best an employer can implement the requirements of Regulations and ensure that they fulfil their legal duties. While ACOPs do not have the full force of the law in the same way as regulations, they have greater 'weight' than guidance and are often referred to as 'semi-legislative' in nature. In practice this means that, if an employer chooses not to comply with the provisions of an ACOP, but to implement the law in an alternative way, in a legal situation the onus will be on that employer to show that they have complied with the law, rather than with the prosecuting party to show that they have not, which would be the normal onus of proof otherwise.

Guidance notes: this brings us finally to guidance notes, which accompany some sets of Regulations and/or ACOPs. They provide even greater detail on the practical implementation of the law and, while it is not legally binding on employers to follow such guidance notes, they often provide the most comprehensive, useful and practical advice to employers having been drawn up by experts in the particular area they cover. They usually also have the additional benefit of being written in much plainer language. So, to continue with the above example of provision of sanitary conveniences in the Workplace Regulations, the ACOP to Regulation 20 goes on to specify the numbers of water closets and washing stations that should be provided in relation to numbers of staff using them.

Legal duties: health and safety law uses different phraseology to denote the level of legal duty imposed by a particular provision and these can essentially be divided into absolute and qualified duties. Where the law imposes an absolute duty on an employer the terms 'must' or 'shall' are usually used. This means that an employer must do exactly what is set out. There is no flexibility in this respect. For example, Regulation 8 of the Workplace (Health, Safety and Welfare) Regulations 1992, sets out that:

Every workplace shall have suitable and sufficient lighting.

However, many of the duties under health and safety law are not absolute, but qualified. This is usually denoted by the use of phrases such as 'an employer shall, so far as is reasonably practicable, ensure...' For example:

The following paragraph of Regulation 8 of these Regulations goes on to say:

The lighting mentioned in paragraph 1 shall, so far as is reasonably practicable, be by natural light.

In these circumstances, it is vital that a manager understands what should be taken into account when judging whether or not it is 'reasonably practicable' for them to do or not do something. This term has appeared in various pieces of legislation over many years, hence there is a legal definition to help, which has resulted from case law. Essentially – although it could be referred to, in its crudest terms, as a cost-benefit analysis – an employer must look at the 'cost' – in time, money and effort – of avoiding a particular risk or implementing a particular requirement and then set this against the level of risk posed by not addressing the hazard or problem. It can only be justifiable not to address the risk if there is found to be a 'gross disproportion' between the two, the risk being insignificant in relation to the costs of avoiding it.

Employers' legal duties

Duties under HASAWA

As the overarching Act under which the specific legal requirements are introduced, HASAWA places a wide range of general duties on employers, as well as imposing some legal responsibilities on other parties such as manufacturers, owners of premises and employees. Under the Act, employers have duties towards all those using their premises and in healthcare establishments this will include patients, visitors, voluntary and self-employed workers as well as employees, to whom the greatest duties apply.

Section 2 of the Act sets out the 'general duties' that employers have towards their employees. These cover all the basic areas which contribute to a safe and healthy working environment including the provision of relevant information and training; a safe place of work; safe working systems; adequate welfare facilities; a written health and safety policy and a Safety Committee where it is requested by safety representatives. We will return to the last two of these later in the chapter and for more information on the Act itself, please refer to the further reading and references sections at the end of the chapter.

Duties under other regulations

As a result of the development of a European-wide market for goods, services and workers, the majority of UK health and safety regulations have emanated from European Union Directives since the 1980s. These set out key elements and standards in specific areas, which are interpreted by member states and incorporated into domestic legislation.

Some of the most important regulations affecting AHPs at work have been introduced as a result of such EU Directives, including the 'Six-Pack', the Working Time Regulations and those covering hazardous substances and the reporting of workplace injuries.

The 'six-pack'

This set of six regulations implemented together in the early 1990s is without doubt one of the most important provisions in UK Health and Safety law, covering a range of duties in specific areas but also containing the regulations which inform employers what is expected of them in relation to managing health and safety in the workplace. The regulations cover:

1 management of health and safety at work regulations and workplace risk assessment
2 manual handling operations
3 workplace regulations
4 display screen equipment (DSE)
5 personal protective equipment
6 work equipment.

Each of the six is summarised briefly below, with particular attention given to the management regulations, due to their particular relevance in relation to risk assessment.

The management of health and safety at work regulations and workplace risk assessment

Usually referred to as the 'management regs', these first came into effect in 1993 and were last updated in 1999.[5] They have particular significance as the regulations which spell out an employer's explicit duties to conduct risk assessments of all their work activities and use these assessments as the basis of preventing and controlling risk. They contain a number of other important provisions, including procedures for dealing with serious and imminent danger, working in premises owned by another employer, the provision of information and training to employees and specific regulations relating to pregnant workers, the last of which we shall return to later. Managers may need to access the full regulations and the reference is given at the end of the chapter; however, for these purposes we will be concentrating on the risk assessment provisions, in Regulations 3 and 4.

The law requires employers to carry out a general risk assessment in order to determine whether there are any hazards in their workplace and what, if any, risks are posed by those hazards. They are also required to take action to prevent or – if that is not possible – control those risks; the results of implementation of such control measures should be monitored and reviewed at appropriate regular intervals to ensure that they remain sufficient. Control measures should aim first to avoid a risk entirely or, if that is not possible, to combat it at source. If that cannot be achieved, the hazard should be isolated and protective equipment should be provided as the main control measure as a last resort.

Risk assessment in practice

Risk assessment is a phrase which often strikes fear into the hearts of those who think they may have responsibility for conducting them and this is because it has been over-complicated. The assessment of risks at work is an extremely important process but does not need to be a difficult one; common sense and the practical experience of both managers and all relevant staff, goes a long way towards getting it right, when coupled with the appropriate training. This does not mean, of course, that one risk assessor can or should know everything and there may be times when it is necessary to call on someone from outside the department for their particular expertise, for example when assessing risks of stress or asbestos exposure. The HSE also provides a number of pieces of guidance for managers conducting risk assessments, including '5 steps to risk assessment'.[6]

Healthcare establishments, whether in the NHS or outside, are usually comparatively large organisations and the process of assessing and eliminating risk is a more highly-developed one than in a much smaller organisation. A typical NHS Trust will have a manager with overall responsibility for health and safety, sometimes known as the 'Risk Manager', as well as a number of managers with delegated health and safety responsibilities in their own areas or departments. AHP managers will often themselves be trained risk assessors with overall responsibility for co-ordinating risk assessments in their department, usually assisted by a number of other senior staff.

There is a great deal of variation in the way in which organisations fulfil their risk assessment obligations; this variation extends to the number of risk assessors appointed to assist the employer with this duty, how senior those staff members are, the exact nature of the training given to ensure they are 'competent' for these purposes, how often risk assessments are reviewed and how they are planned. As a result, it is almost impossible to give a recipe for this as AHP managers need to become familiar with the way in which the organisation in which they are a manager chooses to organise in this area. For example, in one workplace a risk assessment may cover all the relevant hazards in the work area being looked at while in another, assessments may be topic-based, focusing on a single issue, such as manual handling, stress or risks of violence.

Organisations will normally have their own standard documentation for use when undertaking risk assessments; whilst there is considerable variation amongst them, they should include:

Box 10.1 Risk assessment documentation requirements.

- assessment of risk, consequences and level of risk – for example – low, medium, high
- all staff affected, including highlighting groups that may be disproportionately affected, such as pregnant staff and people with disabilities
- any other people affected, such as patients and visitors
- the work environment
- relevant legal standards
- emergency procedures in place
- training
- control measures already in place
- further control measures recommended
- review date and signature of competent person – risk assessor
- the date of the assessment
- brief information regarding the task, area or job being assessed
- actual and potential hazards

What is a hazard and what is a risk?

Risk assessment can be made more difficult by the confusion that often exists in relation to these terms. For these purposes:

- **a hazard** is something with the potential to cause harm
- **a risk** is the likelihood that the harm will arise from the hazard
- **the extent of risk** includes the number of people who might be affected and/or the severity of the consequences.

Example:

- **hazard**: a floor surface which becomes slippery when wet
- **risk**: slips, trips and falls
- **extent of risk**: will include how often and in what circumstances the floor becomes wet and therefore slippery; the number of people using that area of floor; and other factors which could affect the severity of harm, such as the area of flooring being at the top of a flight of stairs or close to a dangerous piece of machinery and so on.

Another regulation contained in the management regulations which is likely to affect AHP managers is the situations where employees work in premises not owned by their own employer. This is increasingly common in the AHP services with staff working in a wide range of settings outside the Trust. Locations might include GP practices and health centres, schools, local authority residential homes and day centres, local authority and private nursing homes and many more.

In such circumstances, Regulation 12 of the regulations requires the 'host' employer to provide visiting employees with comprehensive information about any potential risks to their health, and the local health and staff side procedures, including evacuation. It is important to note that the employer retains their overall duty of care for their own employees in these situations.

The manual handling operations regulations 1992/1999

Manual handling is particularly prominent amongst potential causes of harm or injury in the health services accounting for more than half of all reported accidents, with almost two-thirds of these involving patient handling. Handling is inherent in the work of many AHPs, involving the handling of both patients and other loads. The Manual Handling Operations Regulations[7] define manual handling as:

> Any transporting or supporting of a load and require employers to avoid manual handling involving a risk of injury whenever possible. Where this is not possible or appropriate, a full risk assessment must be conducted and suitable control measures put in place to reduce risk to an acceptable level.

The regulations go into considerable detail regarding this, which includes for example, the rehabilitation of patients and also require employers to provide employees with information and training relating to manual handling.

There is a range of guidance documents available in this area and managers may need to access particular ones from time to time. Visiting the HSE website and those of the AHPs is the best way to access the most up-to-date information; details of these are given at the end of the chapter.

The workplace (health, safety and welfare) regulations 1992

This part of the 'six-pack' covers a wide range of issues relating to the physical working environment[8] and is very useful to managers dealing with common problems, such as lack of space or inadequate changing and toilet facilities. Topics addressed by these regulations include:

Box 10.2 Workplace regulations (1992) topics.

- ventilation
- temperature
- lighting
- space
- sanitary conveniences
- washing facilities
- supply of drinking water
- changing facilities
- suitable and sufficient seating
- rest areas
- facilities for eating meals.

For further details, managers should refer to their local policies or to the regulations themselves.

Display screen equipment

The Health and Safety (Display Screen Equipment) Regulations 1992[9] have become increasingly relevant to AHPs over the last decade and a half since their introduction, with increasing computer use in healthcare. These regulations set minimum standards for the provision, design and use of workstations for employees deemed as 'significant users'.

For these purposes, a 'user' is defined as someone who uses display screen equipment as a significant part of their normal work and the guidance to the regulations defines this further as someone who uses a VDU for continuous spells of an hour or more at a time. The regulations require all workstations to comply with the provisions. Workers who are significant users have additional provisions relating to them, including the right to free eye tests on request, the right to breaks from DSE use and provision of training and information. As with the other 'six-pack' regulations, these provisions are based on the assessment and control of risks.

The personal protective equipment regulations 1992[10]

These regulations cover the provision of protective equipment to employees in situations where it has not been possible to control risks adequately by other means. They also set standards for the provision of such equipment, for example that it must allow the wearer to conduct their job properly, must be stored suitably and be available in a range of sizes.

Work equipment

Finally, in the 'six-pack', the Provision and Use of Work Equipment Regulations 1992[11] control the selection, use and maintenance of all types of machinery, tools and equipment. Based on risk assessment, they require work equipment to be suitable for the task, properly maintained and in good repair. As with the other regulations, employees must be provided with relevant instruction and training in the use of the equipment provided.

While the 'six-pack' is widely viewed as a particularly important set of health and safety provisions, there are many other regulations which will also impact on managers in the AHPs. It is not possible to cover them all here, but a few of the most relevant are outlined below.

The control of substances hazardous to health regulations 1999[12]

These regulations, commonly referred to as COSHH, place an obligation on employers to assess the risks which may arise from exposure to any hazardous substances in their workplace; the regulations also list the substances which have particular defined permissible occupational exposure levels and the list is updated from time to time to ensure that it remains relevant and comprehensive. As with regulations that have already been considered, employers are required to eliminate the hazardous substance whenever possible or to use a less harmful substitute; other control measures may be considered where that is not practicable and protective equipment used as the control measure only if there are no other more effective means to combat the risk.

The working time regulations 1998[13]

The introduction of these ground-breaking regulations for the first time sought to apply some legal parameters to working hours and rest provisions in the UK. Managers needing fuller information should refer to the regulations themselves or the guidance documents available from AHP organisations including the Chartered Society of Physiotherapy.[14] Healthcare organisations must also have organisation-wide policies relating to working time, which may be supplemented by policies at departmental level where needed, for example in relation to 'on-call' systems for groups such as physiotherapists or radiographers.

Some of the key provisions of the regulations include:

Box 10.3 Working time regulations – key points.

- the right to a minimum of four weeks paid holiday per year
- a limit of 48 hours on the average working week
- the right to an in-work rest break – in the health services this right is almost always already superseded by the contractual right to a break or breaks
- a minimum daily continuous rest break of 11 hours
- a minimum weekly continuous rest break of 24 hours or 48 hours in a fortnight.

Where rest requirements are breached, for example by the need to provide a night-time 'on-call' service using staff who have already been working during the day, an employer is obliged to provide 'compensatory rest' within a particular time frame. Once again, local policies should set out the arrangements clearly and managers should refer to these.

The Reporting of Injuries, Diseases and Dangerous Occurrences regulations (RIDDOR) 1995

These reporting requirements, usually known simply as RIDDOR, are important for AHP managers to be familiar with, in order to ensure that relevant events and absences from work are reported not only internally but also to the HSE, as required by this law. Accurate reporting is vital in order for the HSE to establish which work activities and which hazards are causing injuries and other forms of ill-health across the UK working population; it is widely accepted that there is currently a significant level of under-reporting leading to inaccuracies in the picture of work-related ill-health.

Managers should refer to their local policies to ensure that they are clear about their own responsibilities for reporting, but the law essentially provides that the following should be reported:

- work-related accidents involving a fatality or major injury – as defined in the regulations – to any person, including a member of the public

- work-related accidents involving an employee which lead to them being unable to work for more than three consecutive days – including where the absence has been caused by an act of physical violence
- particular potentially dangerous occurrences, as set out in the regulations
- particular 'notifiable' diseases, as prescribed under the Department of Work Pensions Industrial Injuries Scheme.

Managing health and safety in practice

Having outlined the overall legal framework in health and safety and some of the main relevant regulations, we can turn to what this means for managers in practical terms.

The general health and safety policy for the organisation, along with any additional departmental health and safety policies should outline an employer's approach to health and safety and how they intend to control workplace risks and ensure that workers are healthy and safe while at work. The HSC has issued guidance for employers on drawing up policy statements and it is important that managers are familiar with their own employer's general health and safety policy or policies, as well as with specific policies across a range of related matters, including:

Box 10.4 Items to be included in organisational health and safety policies.

- moving and handling
- risk assessment
- pregnant workers
- stress at work
- bullying at work
- working time
- sickness absence
- violence and aggression at work
- lone working
- fire safety and emergency procedures
- infection risks at work and infection control
- latex
- needlesticks and other 'sharps'
- ionising radiation
- COSHH.

All workplace health and safety policies should be monitored, reviewed and updated regularly. They should take into account the whole of an organisation's workforce, including those who work off-site or at night, should be easily available to and widely-known by staff.

Health and safety responsibilities of AHP managers

The degree of legal health and safety responsibility that an organisation delegates to its managers will vary from one organisation to another and with the level and scope of each manager's role within their organisation. Employers should provide all managers with information which makes their role and level of responsibility clear to them.

Departmental or service managers will usually have a number of health and safety responsibilities. Box 10.5 lists the most common:

Box 10.5 Managers' health and safety responsibilities.

- keeping the accident book and records
- reporting matters required under RIDDOR to the health and safety manager for external reporting
- accompanying safety representatives during inspections when requested and taking the required action afterwards
- drawing up any department-level policies on health and safety matters
- co-ordinating and conducting risk assessments and ensuring the recommended control measures are implemented
- meeting safety representatives to discuss health and safety problems or issues and implementing necessary action
- ensuring that all staff receive mandatory and other relevant training at appropriate intervals
- identifying trained first aiders for the department
- identifying staff members to assist with health and safety duties, such as risk assessment
- liaising with occupational health as necessary.

Working with safety representatives

Most AHP managers will work in organisations where trade unions are recognised for collective bargaining and consultation purposes. Where this is the case, there will almost always be accredited trade union safety representatives in place and their roles and rights are set out in the Safety Representatives and Safety Committees Regulations 1996[15] also known as the 'Brown Book'. Even in workplaces that do not recognise trade unions, such as some independent sector organisations, workers have the right to be consulted over health and safety matters and to appoint representatives for this purpose; these rights are set out in a separate piece of legislation.[16]

While it is vital that safety representatives and managers work closely together on workplace health and safety issues, the role and rights of representatives are distinct from the role and legal duties of employers and those that employers appoint to assist them in fulfilling their legal health and safety obligations; it is important that this distinction is clear and understood by managers, safety representatives and other staff to avoid confusion.

The role of a safety representative is to represent the views and interests of employees and they should be elected by the group of members that they are going to represent. As they are appointed by trade unions, they can only represent the members of the union that accredits them following their election. So for example, in a joint therapy department including physiotherapy, occupational therapy, and speech and language therapy there would be safety representatives from at least three unions.

The main unions that AHPs belong to and will therefore elect safety representatives (and stewards) from are:

*   AMICUS for speech and language therapists
*   the British Dietetics Association for dietitians (BDA)
*   the British Orthoptic Society for orthoptists (BIOS)
*   the Chartered Society of Physiotherapy for physiotherapists and physiotherapy assistants (CSP)
*   the Society of Chiropodists and Podiatrists (SCP)
*   the Society of Radiographers for radiographers and allied workers (SOR)
*   UNISON for clerical staff, occupational therapists, some speech and language therapists and some occupational therapy and physiotherapy assistants.

Once elected and accredited by the relevant trade union, safety representatives have certain legal rights as set out in the 'Brown Book'. Some of the key rights include:

Box 10.6 Key rights of health and safety representatives.

*   to be paid for time off to attend relevant union training and to fulfil their main functions. This applies to part-time and full-time staff equally
*   to represent members on health and safety matters, problems and grievances
*   to investigate potential hazards and accidents
*   to investigate health and safety complaints by members
*   to make representations to the employer – via managers – in relation to such investigations
*   to carry out inspections
*   to meet HSE inspectors and receive information from them when they visit or at other relevant times
*   to attend the Safety Committee – where one exists – or to request one to be set up if it does not
*   to have access to certain facilities, such as a notice board, use of a confidential telephone and other means of communicating with members, such as e-mail and the intranet
*   to be consulted over all matters which could have a substantial impact on the health and safety of members.

Workplace inspections

Even though it is the role and legal right of safety representatives to conduct inspections of the workplace, managers are often invited to attend at least some inspections and this method of working together is usually an extremely efficient and effective means of dealing with workplace hazards.

Safety representative's rights allow them to inspect all areas in which their members work at least every three months or more often if there has been a substantial change in working conditions or an accident or dangerous incident. Safety representatives can carry out their inspections alone but it is usually more effective if the safety representative and manager tour the department/work areas together, although this should not preclude members from having time alone to talk to their safety representative about any issues that they need to discuss in confidence. A joint inspection allows both parties to see any hazard or problem which comes to light and to discuss the options for remedial action; as the manager is responsible for organising such remedial action this is an efficient way of addressing problems. In addition, managers are often asked to undertake health and safety audits in their departments and there is a degree of overlap between the areas looked at during such an audit and during an inspection.

The law gives safety representatives the right to conduct inspections at three-monthly intervals, this can cause considerable time pressures, particularly as the way in which healthcare is delivered has changed and diversified so much over the last decade or so. At a time when AHPs tended to be based in one central department or base three-monthly intervals were realistic; however, with staff now based in smaller groups or alone in a much wider variety of workplaces, not all of which are under the complete control of the employer and with a larger variety of working patterns and hours, this has become more difficult. However, there are a number of ways of addressing this, including making sure that there are sufficient safety representatives so that the workload is shared appropriately and drawing up basic checklists so staff in outlying or small premises or clinics can also do their own mini-inspections.

Once the safety representative and manager have either conducted an inspection together or discussed an inspection, a record should be made of the actions that need to be taken; this should include, who is taking the action and the deadline for completion, assisting both safety representatives and managers to review and monitor progress to ensure that workplace hazards have been adequately addressed.

Safety committees

The proper constitution and functions of workplace safety committees are set out in the 'Brown Book' previously referred to. There should be one overarching safety committee covering the whole organisation and this body has the important responsibility of discussing and agreeing organisation-wide policies relating to employee health and safety, as well as highlighting problems and trends in areas such as accidents or absences.

The committee should be made up of trade union safety representatives – the staff side – and managers with relevant roles in the organisations, for example the health and safety manager and those responsible for infection control, manual handling, fire, security. The committee should meet as often as it needs to conduct its business effectively and bi-monthly is a common frequency.

In addition to this overarching safety committee, many organisations have smaller committees to supplement the main one and deal with areas specific to one locality or base or a particular group of staff. So, for example, it is relatively common for a therapies manager to have regular meetings with all the safety representatives in the departments they manage in order to discuss general issues and any that are specific to that group, which might include 'on-call' arrangements or lone working during extended hours clinics.

Common health and safety hazards and problems

Having looked at the law and the workplace structures and arrangements to protect staff and foster a positive health and safety culture, it is also important to consider a number of the most common hazards affecting members of the AHPs. It is beyond the scope of this chapter to consider them all, but a few are introduced.

Pregnant staff

Although pregnancy is not a hazard in itself, some aspects of work may pose a hazard to pregnant staff. The AHPs include a large proportion of women workers and as a result, a considerable proportion of them will be pregnant and returning from maternity leave at some point during their working lives. It is therefore an issue which almost all AHP managers will come across from time-to-time.

Pregnant staff have particular protection in law and the employer's duties toward new and expectant mothers are set out in the Management of Health and Safety at Work Regulations 1999.[5] The relevant regulations (16–8) require employers to undertake specific risk assessments for pregnant workers, taking account of all the risks which may affect them; the risks should first be assessed when the staff member notifies the manager that they are pregnant and then represented at regular intervals to ensure that any adaptations or other control measures remain sufficient and appropriate as the pregnancy progresses.

It is impossible to be prescriptive about the risks which may occur due to the wide variety of work undertaken, but some common areas to consider include:

* manual handling, including lifting and working in awkward postures
* 'on-call', night and weekend working
* working in hot conditions, such as some splinting areas or hydrotherapy pools
* work involving driving, which may be difficult for some women in the later stages of pregnancy
* exposure to some infection risks
* exposure to ionising and non-ionising radiation.

Once a risk assessment has been conducted, any control measures deemed necessary to avoid risk should be implemented without delay. In the very rare circumstances where it is not possible for an employer to modify work or re-deploy a member of staff to an area which is safe for them to work in when pregnant, employees have the right to be suspended on full pay on medical grounds until the beginning of their maternity pay.

All organisations should have a policy relating to the health, safety and risk assessment of pregnant staff and new mothers returning to work and managers should make sure that they are familiar with these. A number of allied health organisations also have guidance in this area and the relevant website contact details are given after the conclusion of this chapter.

Musculoskeletal disorders

Musculoskeletal disorders remain a major cause of work-related ill-health across the UK, prompting the HSE to identify this as a priority area following publication of the Revitalising Health and Safety Strategy[17] and Securing Health Together long-term occupational health strategy[18] in 2000.

Members of the AHPs exhibit a wide range of musculoskeletal injuries and other symptoms, reflecting the diversity of the work they do and specialities they practise in. Not surprisingly, spinal pain – low back, upper back and neck pain –

is the most common followed by upper limb symptoms, including wrist and hand pain. Symptoms in other body parts and joints are less common although they may exist in clusters in particular areas of work such as knee pain amongst paediatric therapists, caused by prolonged kneeling.

Box 10.7 Case studies.

In 2005, the Chartered Society of Physiotherapy conducted a major study into musculoskeletal disorders in 10% of its members – including physiotherapists, physiotherapy assistant and students.[19]

Despite twelve years having elapsed since the introduction of the manual handling regulations, the survey disclosed some worrying statistics:

- over the course of their careers more than 66% of CSP members will suffer from a musculoskeletal disorder
- 58% of members reported symptoms in the last year
- 25% reported symptoms in the last week
- 43% reported more than one episode of symptoms, whether recurrence of the same problem or new problems
- almost 50% of respondents had experienced low back pain, the most prevalent injury or symptom in this AHP group
- a particularly worrying finding was that members were at their most vulnerable to injury when young and/or new to the profession, with 58% being below 30 years when they experienced their most serious or significant problem.

The Society of Radiographers has also looked into this area amongst its members:

- a survey in 2000 showed that 70% of radiographers and 79% of sonographers reported symptoms of pain they believed to be work related[20]
- a further study of 300 sonographers found the prevalence of musculoskeletal disorder amongst sonographers to be 89%[21]
- a 2002 Society of Radiographers study into the causes of musculoskeletal disorders in sonographers found that poor ergonomics, poor posture, lack of rest breaks and inadequate equipment design were key factors contributing to injury. The same study found that whilst 66% of employers carried out risk assessments after an injury was reported, only a minority of employers were carrying out preventative risk assessments prior to any injuries.[22]

In approaching this area, with a view to preventing musculoskeletal disorders, managers will be able to follow the general risk assessment guidance in the Management of Health and Safety at Work Regulations and the specific and detailed guidance on risk assessment in this area in the Manual Handling Operations Regulations; including information on the working environment, the load being handled, individual capabilities and the task as well as guidance on information and training requirements. All organisations are likely to have a detailed policy covering moving and handling and one or more manual handling and/or back care advisers in post to give specialist guidance and assistance.

Manual Handling should form an integral part of induction training thereby ensuring that new staff are familiar with the organisation's policy in this area from the start of their employment. They should be informed where manual handling equipment is stored, when mechanical aids are indicated and should also understand the employer's policy in the important area of handling people for rehabilitation and treatment purposes. Managers may also wish to refer to the HSE website for further guidance on moving and handling issues and to the various AHP organisations' own publications.

Work-related stress

Second only to musculoskeletal disorders, stress at work is now the major cause of work-related ill health and absence from work in the UK economy and healthcare is one of the worst affected sectors.

The huge increase in work-related stress in recent years can be attributed to many factors including a greater awareness of the issue and its symptoms, a change in the nature and intensity of work, constant organisational change and its consequent insecurity, financial instability and many other factors so common in the health services today.

For further information managers should refer to Chapter 11, which introduces the HSE Management Standards, intended to assist managers in assessing and addressing risks of stress at work. Organisations should have a policy in place which aims to prevent stress at work and which sets out the employer's approach in this area.

Bullying at work

As a significant cause of stress at work bullying is not uncommon in healthcare organisations, as in other parts of the economy. It takes a wide range of forms and can be one of the most challenging health and safety and employment issues that managers will ever have to face, often entailing situations where alleged perpetrator and victim are in the same department or work area.

As with all other management issues, managers should look to the organisation's senior management and human resources functions for support and guidance when dealing with bullying; the organisation should have both a policy statement and procedure in this area, which ensures that all such problems are addressed consistently, within a policy framework. Organisations should take bullying extremely seriously and have a zero tolerance approach to tackling it.

Many AHP organisations and trade unions have their own guidance in this area but managers may also wish to refer to an NHS Employer's publication[23] which can be accessed along with campaign materials to support Ban Bullying at Work Day and a wide range of other health and safety information available via their website at www.nhsemployers.org.

Violence and aggression and lone working

These two linked issues are particularly important in healthcare and in any work situation where staff come into contact with members of the public, particularly when they are in stressful or worrying situations; such as awaiting a diagnosis, visiting a sick relative or receiving unwelcome news about how long they may have to wait for an appointment.

Work-related violence and aggression takes many forms, from physical attack to threats and verbal abuse and managers should always be aware that such incidents arising from work do not necessarily occur during working hours or even on the employer's premises; this should be taken into account when assessing risks of violence and aggression.

There is no specific 'law' relating to violence and aggression, which should be addressed as part of the employer's responsibilities to assess, prevent or control all risks to staff health and safety. There is, however, a wealth of guidance available from the HSE, professional organisations and trade unions and from the NHS Employers organisation. Many managers will remember the prominent 'Zero Tolerance' campaign in this area which began in the late 1990s.

It is common for this area to be addressed at induction or other health and safety workplace training with some organisations including it in their mandatory training requirements. The focus of such training should be on recognising and de-escalating potentially violent and aggressive situations and making sure it is possible to leave the incident, rather than resorting to self-defence, which was popular in the past. The NHS Counter Fraud and Security Management Service has also done work in this area which managers may wish to refer to at www.cfsms.nhs.uk.

Lone working is often considered to be a linked issue as one of the major risks associated with working alone is the risk of abuse or attack. Lone working has always existed in the provision of healthcare but is becoming ever more prevalent with changes to the ways in which AHPs provide their services. Members of the professions increasingly work in a wider range of previously atypical work settings in their local communities, alone or in small groups with flexible hours and patterns of work. It is, therefore, vital that Trusts and other healthcare establishments have effective policies to assess and control the risks that arise from working alone, including not only risks of violence but also manual handling and the stress that can arise from working in isolation.

Managers should refer to their employer's policies in this area, but will probably also need to supplement this with a policy for the groups of staff that they manage. Once again, useful guidance can be obtained through the websites of the organisations representing AHPs.

Other health and safety hazards

The issues outlined represent a few of the many health and safety issues facing managers in the AHPs and those that they manage. There are many important specific hazards which may affect some groups more than others which are not covered in this chapter, these include:

- latex and latex allergy
- hazards in hydrotherapy pools
- ionising and non-ionising radiation
- solvents and other hazardous substances
- infection risks
- noise
- dust

- needlestick injuries – see also www.needlestickforum.net for information from the Safer Needles Network.

Managers facing these issues should consult their own employer's policy if one exists or refer to the relevant AHP organisations for further information.

Managing sickness absence and return to work

Although there are many reasons why a member of staff may be on sick leave at any particular time, dealing with sickness absence is in part a health and safety issue as well as a general employment matter. This is both because ill health arising out of an accident or incident at work may lead directly to a period of absence and also because periods of absence not related to work may have health and safety implications particularly at the point when a member of staff is returning from sick leave.

All organisations are likely to have policies which set out sick leave and sick pay entitlements and also offer managers guidance on how sickness absence should be recorded, monitored and managed. They should also make managers aware of other benefits available to people off work with work-related problems, such as the NHS Pensions Agency Temporary Injury Allowance and Permanent Injury Benefit and the Department of Work and Pensions Industrial Injuries Disablement Benefit.

Local policies should also include guidance on issues such as how often staff should call in when off sick, what advice the organisation gives about managers initiating contact with staff on sick leave, when managers should make a referral to the occupational health department and to whom should doctors' certificates be submitted. This sort of basic procedural guidance is useful and helps managers to treat all staff consistently and equitably in this respect.

In recent years there has been a growing realisation of the cost to the UK economy which results from the comparatively low proportion of UK workers who return successfully to work following a significant or lengthy period of sick leave in comparison with other European countries. Taking stock of practice in other countries, more flexible approaches to return to work and rehabilitation have developed. Thus, most local sickness absence policies will now make specific reference to phased and supported return to work periods, with organisations being far more open to modifying both duties and working hours to enable an earlier return to the workplace or even avoid someone needing to be off work in the first place.

Managers are usually responsible for co-ordinating a member of staff's return to work following a significant absence; this often involves a number of meetings with the staff member and often their representative – steward or safety – as well as HR adviser if needed, to agree the details of the phased return. It is normally appropriate and necessary to undertake a specific risk assessment in these circumstances to ensure that all aspects of the member's usual work have been considered prior to their return. The other department that is often involved and can be extremely useful in this situation is the occupational health department, which will have staff with particular knowledge and expertise in the interface between work and health.

Managers can refer to a number of pieces of good practice guidance in this area, including those drawn up by NHS Employers, HSE and the relevant trade unions and professional organisations.

Managing health and safety successfully

The successful management of workplace health and safety is a complex matter involving the law, good practice guidance, local policies and general management experience and skills. Both the Healthcare Commission and the NHS Litigation Authority have recently set and/or updated standards in this area and these are summarised with the relevant references given for further information. Also outlined is some of the HSE's own guidance on successful health and safety management.

'Standards for Better Health' and health and safety

The Department of Health core and developmental Standards for Better Health published in 2004 contain standards on health and safety including ones on incident reporting, risk management, safe working environments, hospital cleanliness and hygiene and the management of violence and aggression. Healthcare organisations providing care to NHS patients are required to comply with the core standards and be working towards achieving the developmental standards. The process is one of self assessment and Trust Boards are responsible for signing a public declaration to state whether the Trust has met the standards or not. The Healthcare Commission is responsible for checking an organisation's performance against the standards, which feed into the annual ratings. Further information on the standards can be found at www.healthcarecommission.org.uk.

NHS litigation authority risk management standards for trusts

The NHS Litigation Authority, which is effectively the NHS's insurance body, introduced new Risk Management Standards for Acute Trusts in 2007. The standards which were previously focused on clinical risk and known as the CNST, specifically make reference to work related stress policies; policies and strategies on reduction of violence and aggression and bullying and harassment. Within the standards there are three levels to be achieved, the top level can be achieved when Trusts show that policy and practice is 'embedded' and actively monitored. Trusts that meet the standards will be subject to a discount in the amount of money they contribute to the insurance scheme. The higher the level they meet the more the discount, so there are clear financial incentives as well as the legal and moral duties, to have effective policies/strategies in place.

The information on what level a Trust has met will also feed into the Healthcare Commission annual health check, which feeds into performance ratings, and will give the Healthcare Commission data on whether Trusts are meeting the Department of Health's Standards for Better Health relating to safe and secure environment. More information on the NHSLA Risk Management Standards for Trusts can be found at www.nhsla.com/RiskManagement/CnstStandards/.

Further guidance from the HSE

The Health and Safety Executive identify five steps to successful health and safety management:[24]

- Step 1: set your policy
- Step 2: organise your staff
- Step 3: plan and set standards
- Step 4: measure your performance
- Step 5: learn from experience – audit and review.

These have been identified as a source of best practice by the Healthcare Commission in assisting Trusts to meet the developmental standards under Standards for Better Health.[25] These five steps can be implemented at a local departmental level as well as a Trust wide level. The steps and examples of local implementation are:

Step 1: set your policy

A Trust-wide health and safety policy will be set at an organisation-wide level, however it may be necessary to have local policies where specific hazards and risks are identified.

Checklist for managers

When setting and reviewing policies the following questions should be asked:

- are departmental policies clear and written down?
- what did the department achieve in health and safety last year?
- how much is being spent on health and safety and are you getting value for money?
- how much money is being lost by not managing health and safety?
- does your policy prevent injuries, reduce losses and really affect the way you work?

Step 2: organise your staff

The HSE point out that to make a health and safety policy effective you need to get staff involved and committed. This is often referred to as a positive health and safety culture. There are four 'Cs' to achieving this:

Box 10.8 The 4 Cs for a positive health and safety culture.

competence – recruitment, training, supervision of to ensure competency of staff and access to competent advisors for example, back care/manual handling advisors

control – securing commitment is key and requires top level commitment including leading by example. Local managers and supervisors need to clearly understand their responsibilities and have the time and resources to carry these out

co-operation – consultation is a key aspect of co-operation. Effective consultation with local trade union safety representatives through, for example local health and safety meetings or making health and safety an agenda item at staff meetings is paramount. Involving staff through their trade union representatives in planning and reviewing performance, writing procedures and solving problems will create a positive health and safety culture

communication – managers must provide information about hazards risks and preventative measures to employees, students and contractors, for example agency staff working on the premises, again making health and safety an agenda item on local staff meetings is a way of promoting a positive health and safety message. Anonymised details of departmental accidents and near misses can be communicated at such meetings, including what action has been taken as a result of serious incidents or trends.

Checklist for managers

- Have you allocated responsibilities for health and safety to specific people within the department – are they clear on what they have to do and are they held accountable and suitably remunerated for the extra responsibility?
- Do you consult and involve trade union safety representatives on any changes being planned and decision making and policy development which can affect health and safety?
- Do your staff or any others working in the department for example students on placement or agency staff, have sufficient information about the risks they run and the preventive measures?
- Do you have the right levels of expertise within your department and are your people properly trained?
- Do you need specialist advice from outside and have you arranged and obtained it?

Step 3: plan and set standards

Planning for health and safety involves setting local objectives, identifying hazards, assessing risks, implementing standards of performance and developing a positive safety culture. Planning should provide for:

- identifying hazards, assessing risks and deciding how they can be eliminated or controlled
- complying with the health and safety laws that apply to your organisation
- agreeing health and safety targets with managers, supervisors and trade union safety representatives
- a purchasing and supply policy which takes health and safety into account such as latex in equipment, safer needle devices and ergonomic equipment
- safe systems of work and local rules
- procedures for dealing with serious and imminent danger within a department
- co-operation with other organisations for example between an acute Trust and PCT where premises are shared
- setting standards against which performance can be measured such as benchmarking.

When standard setting it is important that standards are SMART: specific, measurable, achievable, realistic and timed. They should be agreed with local trade union safety representatives.

Checklist for managers

- Do you have a health and safety plan for the department?
- Is health and safety always considered before any new work is started?
- Have hazards been identified and risks assessed?
- Do you communicate and co-operate with other employers/premises' owners where your staff work for example GP surgeries or PCTs?
- Do you have a local plan for dealing with serious or imminent danger such as chemical spillage, fire?
- Are standards put in place?

Step 4: measure your performance

There are two monitoring systems which should be implemented when measuring performance, *active* monitoring and *reactive* monitoring. Active monitoring involves looking for things before they go wrong, for example by carrying out audit or inspections to check whether objectives and standards are being met. Reactive monitoring takes place after things have gone wrong such as investigating injuries and near misses. Trade union safety representatives should be involved in monitoring performance both active and reactive and must be enabled to undertake inspections and investigate accidents and cases of ill health.

Accident and near miss investigation must be thorough and identify the underlying causes which can often be deep rooted within the organisation, rather than just caused by an individual making an error.

Checklist for managers

- Do you know how well you perform in health and safety, for example how do your accident rates compare with other departments?
- Do you have a culture of reporting near misses?
- Do you have accurate records of injuries and ill health within your department?
- Do your accident investigations get to all the underlying causes or do they stop when you find the first person who has made a mistake?
- Do you carry out safety audits and inspections?

Step 5: learn from experience – audit and review

Reactive and Active monitoring provides the information to let you review activities and decide how health and safety performance can be improved.

Checklist for managers

- How do you learn from your mistakes and your successes?
- What action is taken on audit findings?
- What action do you take to implement lessons learnt following accidents and cases of ill health within the department?

Conclusion

In this chapter an overview of the highly complex area of regulating, managing and protecting health, safety and welfare at work has been presented. Health and safety is managed most successfully where its importance is recognised and where it is fully integrated into the mainstream of an organisation's management functions, delivering a positive health and safety culture across the organisation.

A list of suggested further reading is available from a number of organisations, including those representing AHPs and contact details for some are given below.

References

1 www.hse.gov.uk/healthservices/index.htm.
2 www.hse.gov.uk/statistics/industry/healthservices/htm.
3 HSE. *A guide to the Reporting of Injuries, Diseases and Dangerous Occurrences Regulations 1995 L73*. 2nd ed. London: HSE Books; 1999.
4 Health and Safety at Work Act. London: HMSO;1974.
5 HSE. *Management of Health and Safety at Work Regulations 1999. Approved Code of Practice and Guidance L21*. London: HSE Books; 2000.
6 HSE. *5 Steps to Risk Assessment*. London: HSE Books; 2006. www.hse.gov.uk/risk/fivesteps.htm.
7 HSE. *Manual Handling Operations Regulations 1992: Guidance on Regulations L23* 3rd ed. London: HSE Books; 2004.
8 HSE. *Workplace (Health, Safety and Welfare) Regulations 1992. Approved Code of Practice L24*. London: HSE Books; 1993.
9 HSE. *Health and Safety (Display Screen Equipment) Regulations 1992. Miscellaneous Amendments; Regulations 2002. Guidance on Regulations L26*. 2nd ed. London: HSE Books; 2003.
10 HSE. *Personal Protective Equipment at Work Regulations 1992. Guidance on Regulations L25*. London: HSE Books; 2005.
11 HSE. *Provision and Use of Work Equipment Regulations 1998. Approved Code of Practice and Guidance L22*. London: HSE Books; 1998.
12 HSE. *The Control of Substances Hazardous to Health Regulations 2002 (as amended). Approved Code of Practice and Guidance L5*. 5th ed. London: HSE Books; 2005.
13 Sections 1–4 URN No 06.1908A and Sections 5–11 URN No 06/1908B. London: DTI; 2006.
14 Chartered Society of Physiotherapy. Briefing Paper No 22. The Working Time Regulations 1998. London: CSP; 2002.
15 HSE. *Safety Representative and Safety Committees Regulations 1996 L87*. London: HSE Books; 1996.
16 HSE. *A Guide to the Health and Safety (Consultation with Employees) Regulations 1996. Guidance on Regulations. L95*. London: HSE Books; 1996.
17 Department of the Environment, Transport and the Regions. Revitalising Health and Safety: strategy statement. London: The Department of the Environment, Transport and the Regions; 2000.
18 HSE. *Securing Health Together: A long-term occupational health strategy for England, Scotland and Wales. MISC225*. London: HSE Books; 2000.
19 Chartered Society of Physiotherapy. *Work-related musculoskeletal disorders in physiotherapists*. London: CSP; 2005.
20 Arrowsmith I. *The Prevalence of Work-Related Upper Limb Disorders amongst Radiographers*. London: SOR; 2000.
21 Feather C. Work Related Musculoskeletal Disorders: an occupational hazard for sonographers. *Synergy*, 2001; October.
22 Society of Radiographers. *The causes of musculoskeletal injury amongst sonographers in the UK*. London: SOR; 2002.

23 NHS Employers: Bullying and harassment. Available at: www.nhsemployers.org.

24 HSE. *Managing health and safety – five steps to success INDG275*. London: HSE Books; 1998.

25 Healthcare Commission. *Developing the annual health check in 2006/2007 – have your say*. London: Healthcare Commission; 2006.

Further information

Useful websites include:
- www.hse.gov.uk
- www.hsebooks.com/books
- www.tuc.org.uk/h_and_s/
- www.nhsemployers.org
- www.healthcarecommission.org.uk
- www.csp.org.uk – professional body and trade union for physiotherapists, physiotherapy assistant and students
- www.sor.org – professional body and trade union for radiographers, radiotherapists and allied workers
- www.unison.org.uk – trade union for occupational therapists and some other AHPs
- www.feetforlife.org – professional body and trade union for chiropodists and podiatrists
- www.bda.uk.com –professional body and trade union for dieticians
- www.amicustheunion.org – trade union for speech and language therapists and some other AHPs
- www.cot.org.uk – professional body for occupational therapists
- www.rcslt.org – professional body for speech and language therapists
- www.britishorthopticsociety.co.uk – professional body and trade union for orthoptists
- www.bapo.com – professional association for orthotists and prosthetists
- www.cfsms.nhs.uk

Chapter 11

Managing work-related stress

Laura McDonnell

Introduction

The focus of this chapter is an approach which the HSE has developed to manage workplace stress, namely the 'Management Standards'.[1] An overview of the development of the standards is included in the introduction to the management standards – further reading is suggested at the end of the chapter on the evidence-base and the development process. Employers' duties in terms of Health and Safety law and stress, in particular the requirement to carry out a risk assessment, are explained – however, employment law is not covered; see book one in this series, *Managing and Leading in the Allied Health Professions*, Chapter 8 Legal Issues.

The aim of this chapter is to provide managers of Health Professions with practical advice to help them develop a 'suitable and sufficient' risk assessment for stress using the HSE Management Standards as a framework. The HSE has developed a process and tools to accompany the Standards and help managers carry out their risk assessment. How to apply the process and tools is explained, followed by an in-depth case study from one NHS Trust. The HSE recognises that there are other approaches to managing stress at an organisational level therefore the chapter also sets out key elements to look for when deciding whether another approach to managing work-related stress is suitable before concluding with some thoughts on the future direction of the HSE activity in this area.

The approach to tackling work-related stress is predicated on prevention of stress at work by ensuring that good management practices are in place and more importantly are in use. This is known as primary intervention. However, not every 'case' of work-related stress is preventable. Other factors, in particular those outside the workplace and hence beyond the control of managers, do have an effect on employees and those around them while they are at work. Many of the support systems – often known as secondary interventions – designed to help employees who are experiencing work-related stress can also help address non-work causes. The latter approach forms the basis of a campaign by the NHS Employers; more information on this is available on their website.[2]

The HSE focus on the health sector is part of a much broader drive to tackle work-related ill-health in the public sector, following the establishment of a Ministerial Task Force to look at public sector management of sickness absence and return to work.[3] In 2005 the average cost of sickness absence to an NHS Trust in England was £3.8 million – representing a 16% increase on 2004 prices.[4] Since 2000 there has been no significant change in NHS sickness absence rates.[5]

The reasons for sickness absence are complex and include:

- individual factors – such as motivation, personality, past behaviour, sick role
- the 'system' – organisational culture and tolerability, what is legitimate? for example, sickness certification
- non-work factors – life events and family pressures
- work factors – absence, low job satisfaction and adverse features of work
- commitment and involvement – low morale.

A common theme emerging from the HSE initiatives on both stress and sickness absence is that these issues can be tackled effectively by good management practices that promote 'healthy' workplaces.

Introduction to the management standards

In November 2004 the HSE launched the 'Management Standards' which are designed to help organisations take a risk assessment approach to tackling work-related stress. They are supported by an approach that allows measurement of the current situation using surveys and other techniques, promotes active discussion with employees to help understand the practical improvements that can be made and encourages a culture of continuous improvement.

The HSE's overall aim is to reduce the number of employees who go off sick, or who cannot perform well because of stress at work.[6,7] To achieve this the aim is that employers work with employees and their representatives to implement the management standards. This will benefit employees, employers and the organisation as a whole.

All the materials and tools referred to in this chapter, as well as the management standards, are available free of charge from the HSE website:[1] www.hse.gov.uk/stress/standards. The website is regularly updated to reflect the latest knowledge and experience of tackling work-related stress.

What is stress?

There are many definitions of stress. The HSE definition is:

> Stress is the adverse reaction people have to excessive pressures or other types of demand placed on them.[8]

There is a clear distinction between pressure, which can create a 'buzz' and be a motivating factor, and stress, which can occur when this pressure becomes excessive.

It is important to remember that work-related stress is not an illness but if it is prolonged or particularly intense, it can lead to increased problems with ill health.

For example:

- physical effects such as heart disease, back pain, gastrointestinal disturbances and various minor illnesses
- psychological effects such as anxiety and depression.

Stress can lead to other behaviours that are not helpful to health, such as skipping meals, drinking too much caffeine or alcohol and smoking cigarettes ... and it can happen to anyone.

There are likely to be consequences for organisations where work-related stress is prevalent:

- increased sickness absence can lead to a 'domino effect' as remaining staff try to cope with the workload of sick colleagues. This can in turn lead to further sickness absence
- staff who feel stressed but are still at work may not be performing as well as they would otherwise, leading to an increased risk of accidents or mistakes
- staff morale may be reduced
- staff turnover may increase – along with associated costs of recruitment and training
- staff may seek compensation through civil litigation.

There is evidence from staff[9] and patient surveys[10] carried out in the NHS to show that creating a stable, experienced, workforce, reducing turnover and increasing staff satisfaction, creating a more open and fair culture and reducing stress and injury is directly linked to increased patient satisfaction.

How did the management standards come about?

In 2000 the Health and Safety Commission (HSC) agreed a strategy[11] to address this serious occupational health issue. The HSC recognised that action was needed after a report by the HSE estimated that:

- about one in five people said that they found their work either very or extremely stressful
- over half a million people reported experiencing work-related stress at a level they believed had actually made them ill
- work-related stress cost UK employers approximately £353 million to £381 million a year and cost society between £3.7 billion and £3.8 billion a year (1995/96 prices).

Updated figures indicate that each case of stress-related ill health leads to an average of 30.9 working days lost per person per annum.[12]

The strategy was informed by a public consultation exercise[13] conducted by the HSC in 1999 to gather people's views on how best to tackle stress in the workplace. Almost all of the respondents to the consultation exercise agreed that work-related stress was a legitimate health, safety and welfare issue that should be dealt with under the existing UK regulatory framework. Many wanted an ACOP telling them how to go about tackling work-related stress. However, concerns around enforcement and the practicality of recommending specific interventions that would be effective in all circumstances meant that a different, evidence based approach was needed. The HSC did, however, agree to keep the need for an ACOP under review.

Underpinning this new approach to tackling stress at work are the principles that stress management equals good management and that any interventions, if they are to be successful, must address the underlying causes of stress rather than just the symptoms. While the causes of stress at work can often appear complex and difficult they can be managed through the same risk assessment approach used to manage other workplace hazards. It is from this background that the management standards and supporting approach have grown.

Existing health and safety law

Apart from moral and financial considerations, the Health and Safety at Work etc Act 1974[14] requires employers to ensure the health, safety and welfare at work of all their employees – often referred to as the 'duty of care' – so far as is reasonably practicable.

As work-related stress affects the health of employees it falls within the remit of the Act. Therefore, under the Management of Health and Safety at Work Regulations 1999[15] employers are required to carry out, and act, on the findings of risk assessments. In practise, this means considering the risks associated with stress proactively, rather than waiting for problems to arise and then taking action.

It is important to remember that risk assessments are a means to an end, not an end in themselves; they are done to identify and define the hazards and the degree of risk associated with an activity. They should also determine the methods and procedures that should be put in place to address those risks. These procedures then need to be implemented so that the risks are properly controlled and monitored to ensure they have the intended effect.

The concept of 'reasonable practicability' is important as it allows a degree of flexibility into the system, that is, the degree of resource input can be proportional to the degree of risk. It has also created problems when carrying out stress risk assessments – how do employers assess or measure the degree of risk so that they know what is reasonably practicable for them to do?

How do the management standards help?

The HSE believes that the most successful way of managing stress at work is to carry out a risk assessment. By targeting the root causes at an organisational level the HSE believes organisations can prevent pressure from becoming excessive and causing stress.

The management standards provide a framework to help develop a risk assessment for stress. The standards capture the key characteristics and define the culture of an organisation where stress is being managed effectively.

The supporting approach and tools are designed to help employers compare themselves against the standards. An indicator tool highlights the likely key causes of stress in the workplace and provides a way to measure progress in tackling them.

The approach is designed to deal with issues in the workplace affecting most of the people, most of the time. It encourages employers, employees and their representatives to work in partnership and is predicated on the view that the people doing the job are best placed to know what is causing them stress and what can be done about it.

Sickness absence management

It is worth stating at this point that prevention is not the whole answer and even an organisation that is doing everything it reasonably can to manage the risks may still come across individual cases of work-related stress. It is important that organisations also have in place measures to manage sickness absence attributed to workplace stress, that is as part of a wider sickness absence management policy. Guidance on sickness absence management is also available from HSE's website.[16]

So what are the management standards?

The causes of work-related stress can often be traced to the way jobs are designed and managed. There are six management standards, one for each of six key areas of work design - workplace *stressors* - that if not properly managed are associated with poor health and well-being, lower productivity and increased sickness absence.

1 Demands.
2 Control.
3 Support.
4 Relationships.
5 Role.
6 Change.

1 Demands: includes issues like workload, work patterns and the work environment.

> **Box 11.1 Management standards: demands.**
>
> The standard is:
> - employees indicate that they are able to cope with the demands of their jobs
> - systems are in place locally to respond to any individual concerns.

What should be happening/states to be achieved:

- the organisation provides employees with adequate and achievable demands in relation to the agreed hours of work
- people's skills and abilities are matched to the job demands
- jobs are designed to be within the capabilities of employees
- employees' concerns about their work environment are addressed.

2 Control: how much 'say' the person has in the way they do their work.

> **Box 11.2 Management standards: control.**
>
> The standard is:
> - employees indicate that they are able to cope with the demands of their jobs
> - systems are in place locally to respond to any individual concerns.

What should be happening/states to be achieved:

- where possible, employees have control over their pace of work
- employees are encouraged to use their skills and initiative to do their work
- where possible, employees are encouraged to develop new skills to help them undertake new and challenging pieces of work
- the organisation encourages employees to develop their skills

- employees have a say over when breaks can be taken
- employees are consulted over their work patterns.

3 Support: includes the encouragement, sponsorship and resources provided by the organisation, line management and colleagues.

> **Box 11.3 Management standards: support.**
>
> The standard is:
> - employees indicate that they receive adequate information and support from their colleagues and superiors
> - systems are in place locally to respond to any individual concerns.

What should be happening/states to be achieved:

- the organisation has policies and procedures to adequately support employees
- systems are in place to enable and encourage managers to support their staff
- systems are in place to enable and encourage employees to support their colleagues
- employees know what support is available and how and when to access it
- employees know how to access the required resources to do their job
- employees receive regular and constructive feedback.

4 Relationships: includes promoting positive working to avoid conflict and dealing with unacceptable behaviour.

> **Box 11.4 Management standards: relationships.**
>
> The standard is:
> - employees indicate that they are not subjected to unacceptable behaviours, for example bullying at work
> - systems are in place locally to respond to any individual concerns.

What should be happening/states to be achieved:

- the organisation promotes positive behaviours at work to avoid conflict and ensure fairness
- employees share information relevant to their work
- the organisation has agreed policies and procedures to prevent or resolve unacceptable behaviour
- systems are in place to enable and encourage managers to deal with unacceptable behaviour
- systems are in place to enable and encourage employees to report unacceptable behaviour.

5 Role: whether people understand their role within the organisation and whether the organisation ensures that the person does not have conflicting roles.

> **Box 11.5 Management standards: role.**
>
> The standard is:
> - employees indicate that they understand their role and responsibilities
> - systems are in place locally to respond to any individual concerns.

What should be happening/states to be achieved:

- the organisation ensures that, as far as possible, the different requirements it places upon employees are compatible
- the organisation provides information to enable employees to understand their role and responsibilities
- the organisation ensures that, as far as possible, the requirements it places upon employees are clear
- systems are in place to enable employees to raise concerns about any uncertainties or conflicts they have in their role and responsibilities.

6 **Change**: how organisational change – large or small – is managed and communicated in the organisation.

Box 11.6 Management standards: change.

The standard is:
- employees indicate that the organisation engages them frequently when undergoing an organisational change
- systems are in place locally to respond to any individual concerns.

What should be happening/states to be achieved:

- the organisation provides employees with timely information to enable them to understand the reasons for proposed changes
- the organisation ensures adequate employee consultation on changes and provides opportunities for employees to influence proposals
- employees are aware of the probable impact of any changes to their jobs. If necessary, employees are given training to support any changes to their jobs
- employees are aware of timetables for changes
- employees have access to relevant support during changes.

How can the management standards help the risk assessment process?

In this section the toolkit that the HSE has developed for undertaking risk assessments for stress is presented.

Overview of the process

The five steps[17] to carrying out a risk assessment for stress are:

- Step 1: identify the hazards
- Step 2: decide who may be harmed and how
- Step 3: evaluate the risk and take action
- Step 4: record your findings
- Step 5: monitor and review.

The risk assessment process is normally described as a 'Five Step process' however it is a continuous improvement model which does not end at step five!

An alternative way of thinking about the process is as a 'Gap Analysis' where the management standards represent the target for the organisation. Gathering information is aimed at identifying where the organisation is today in terms of performance against the management standards, that is, measuring the gap. Linking problems to solutions is aimed at working with employees to generate interventions to address the issues identified and close the performance gap.

Feedback[18] indicates that it takes about 18 months to complete one cycle of the management standards process. This period comprises up to six months to undertake the risk assessment and put interventions in place and a further year to monitor progress before going back to measure outcomes.

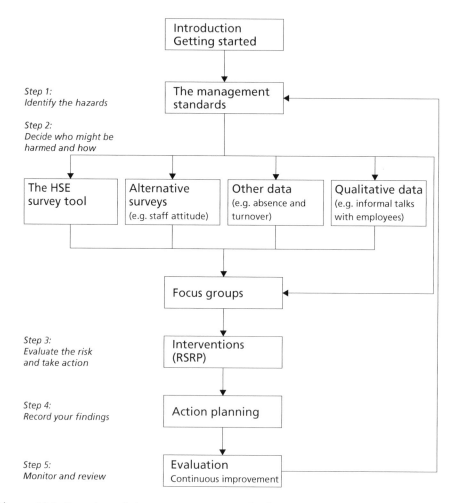

Step 1:
Identify the hazards

Step 2:
Decide who might be harmed and how

Step 3:
Evaluate the risk and take action

Step 4:
Record your findings

Step 5:
Monitor and review

Figure 11.1 Overview of the management standards process.

Before using the management standards

The management standards approach depends very much on establishing and maintaining senior management commitment and staff involvement throughout the process. It is likely that staff will only want to take part in such an initiative if senior management commitment to tackling work-related stress has been clearly demonstrated. It may be helpful to develop an organisational stress policy and get it agreed at Board level. This will underline that senior managers take the issue of stress seriously.

There may be existing policies that are also relevant because they deal with issues that can cause stress, for example, policies on violence and aggression at work, lone working or bullying – the first two are relevant to the standard on demands, which covers the working environment and the latter is relevant to the standard on relationships. It may be necessary to review these as part of the process.

The HSE recommends that the management standards approach is managed in the same way as any other project. Set up a steering group, agree objectives and assign roles and responsibilities to members of the project team. Starting with solid foundations increases the probability of a successful outcome.

Steering group members are typically drawn from:

- senior management
- employee/staff side representative
- trade unions representative
- health and safety manager
- human resources (HR) manager
- occupational health
- line management
- other, for example professional/medical.

The actual membership will be determined by your organisational structures. However, for the project to deliver real improvements and lead to a culture change within the organisation, all employee groups should be involved in the process.

Users of this approach also recommend that individuals are nominated to take on the following key roles:

- **project champion**: to represent the project at Board level, update the Board on progress and ensure the project is adequately resourced. Typically this would be the HR director or facilities director; these post holders have responsibility for sickness absence and/or health and safety policy management and monitoring
- **day-to-day champion**: to take on the role of the 'Project Manager' co-ordinating activities and controlling costs and resources. Typically this would be a Health and Safety manager or in some cases an Occupational Health or HR professional.

The activities of the steering group encompass all usual good project management practices, however, experience shows that there are several areas that the steering group should give particular attention to:

- **senior management commitment**: includes securing resources for the project
- **employee involvement**: the success of the management standards approach depends on effectively engaging employees, from agreeing on what the hazards are to generating action plans. It is important to consider this from the beginning. Involve staff side representatives in any groups which are set up to

do the work, so that the aims are fully understood. If a decision is taken to limit the introduction of the process to only a few departments or sections within the organisation, consideration must be given to how best to communicate this decision to those staff not included

- **resources**: when developing a budget for the project, include time to run the process and for staff to participate. Is there expertise in project management and/or data analysis, or does this need to be bought in?
- **communication**: this is key to the success of the Management Standards approach. It is important to communicate openly and effectively with managers, employees and their representatives throughout the process. Communication needs to be considered and planned from the outset, remembering, quality not quantity. Talking and listening to people is one of the most effective means of communication
- **naming the project**: avoid negative connotations associated with the word 'stress'. Consider a positive title like 'Well Working' or 'Valuing Staff' to emphasise the positive aspects of the approach.

What users have said:

Box 11.7 User views.

- it is vital to achieve one hundred percent commitment from senior management and local management teams
- the 'steering group' is key; choose individuals who are keen to make a contribution and make the project work
- steering group rules include 'egos left at the door'!
- you need a team who can be mutually supportive
- you need a communication strategy – communication is vital
- planning is absolutely critical.

Implementing the management standards

Step 1: understanding the management standards

This step has largely been covered in the earlier part of this chapter, however, if more information is needed about the background, development and evidence underpinning the standards, this is available in the suggestions for further reading and publications referenced at the end of this chapter. Most of this information is available to download free of charge from the HSE website.

Step 2: gathering information

There are two main sources of information that managers can use to discover whether there is a problem with stress in the workplace. Firstly, quantitative data can highlight where an organisation may have a problem and includes:

- sickness absence data
- employee turnover
- exit interviews
- productivity data

- performance reviews
- informal discussions with employees
- surveys
- return to work interviews.

The second source is qualitative data drawn from informal discussions with staff, walk-throughs, focus groups or team meetings. This can help identify where specific problems lie based on what is happening locally. By combining these two types of information managers can gain an overview of their organisation's performance.

Surveys

The validity of self-reporting and questionnaire based surveys is often called into question because they are dependent on how people 'feel' about issues. However, individual perceptions play an important role in predicting stress-related ill health.[19] Therefore, gathering the opinions of employees can be a useful indicator of the health of the organisation and as a part of an overall strategy to identify and address potential sources of stress. A word of caution, however, surveys only give a broad indication of where there may be problems; they cannot specify what is happening locally or what the solution might be. Survey data should always be viewed in context with other quantitative and qualitative data and should be explored through discussions with employees. Surveys should never be used in isolation to develop solutions.

The management standards toolkit, which can be accessed through the HSE website, contains a 35 question survey (the HSE Indicator Tool.) This survey was developed in response to the needs of users and validated through research carried out with employees of Hertfordshire County Council.[20] Organisations can use the indicator tool to get an idea of how they 'shape up' against the standards. The questions cover all six of the stressor areas and highlight areas where an organisation may have problems.

How to assess performance against the management standards

A useful first step is to use existing information to see how your organisation performs. Look for:

- areas of good performance
- existing knowledge of problem areas or 'hotspots'
- correlations between data sources.

Next map the issues in the data across the management standards.

When using the HSE Indicator Tool the accompanying HSE Analysis Tool may also be used. When the results are entered and analysed the tool generates a measurement of organisational performance.

The analysis tool gives an average result for each of the six stressor areas and these are graphically displayed alongside a target figure. The ultimate aim is to be in the top 20% of organisations in tackling work-related stress as assessed by the HSE through modules in two National Omnibus Surveys[21] (nationwide surveys conducted for the UK's Office of National Statistics). If an organisation is currently not achieving the benchmark figure, then an interim figure is also given as a

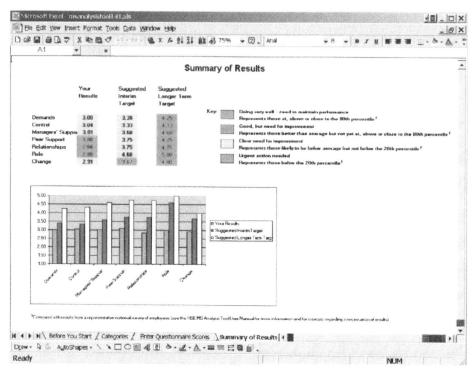

Figure 11.2 Example of the screen display generated by the analysis tool.

'stepping-stone' towards improvement. That is, the HSE supports continuous improvement in stress management.

Whatever data is used, it is still necessary to remember to communicate with employees and their representatives to verify the findings and assess what is happening locally. Explore the facts presented before deciding on solutions, never second guess what the staff response will be.

Box 11.8 Key learning points from users.

- a lot of relevant data was often available but not previously used!
- some data were available through other initiatives for example NHS Annual Staff Survey and Improving Working Lives
- a combination of data gathered centrally and locally (by asking line managers to evaluate staff reviews) has proved helpful when trying to identify triggers
- communicating the survey results has given us an opportunity to celebrate what is working well in the Trust as well as areas where we could improve.

Alternative options to using surveys

Surveys may not be appropriate in teams or departments with relatively few employees. In such cases it may be more appropriate to explore issues related to working conditions in small groups.

Where there are already arrangements in place for engaging and consulting with employees, for example routine team meetings, it would be sensible to use these as an opportunity to discuss potentially stressful issues. Similarly, management meetings can be used to explore potential stressors for this group of staff. However, the composition of such groups needs to be considered together with whether participants are likely to be comfortable discussing these issues in front of each other.

Individual concerns

The surveys and focus groups may identify that some individuals are experiencing problems but the majority of employees are not. The solutions that are developed for the majority of employees may not address the problems experienced by these individuals. However, there is still a duty of care to take steps to protect the health and well-being of these employees too.

It is essential that ways for individual employees to raise their concerns are in place, for example:

- create an environment where employees are encouraged to talk, both formally and informally to their manager or another person in their management chain
- remind employees that they can speak to trade union representatives, health and safety representatives, HR personnel
- encourage employees to talk to someone in the organisation or seek advice from occupational health advisors, or from their GP if they are concerned about their health
- introduce mentoring and other forms of co-worker support
- provide employee assistance (counselling) services.

Where such measures are already in place, be alerted that the management standards approach may trigger an increase in people wanting to use them. This may seem like a cause for concern, however, it may be that employees now feel able to raise the issue and ask for help. It is important that planning takes place for this resource requirement.

Step 3: exploring problems and developing solutions

Each workplace and each worker is different, therefore it is not possible to prescribe one set of solutions for all circumstances. The HSE approach is based on employers, employees and their representatives working in partnership to explore problems and develop solutions. There are many ways of doing this, for example: team briefings, cascade briefings, existing working groups and other staff forums.

A good way is to bring together groups of about six to ten employees as a 'focus group'. Discussions with a selection of employees from a specific work group provides an opportunity to explore the findings from the data gathering step and take into account local challenges. It also allows discussion in a supportive and confidential environment, helping people work together to generate SMART – Specific Measurable Achievable Relevant and Timed – interventions.

Many users have found organising and getting people to attend focus groups one of the more challenging aspects of the management standards approach, particularly where this involves shift workers or 'front line' staff. However, those that have successfully managed to overcome the challenges highlight it as one of the most rewarding parts of the approach.

Box 11.9 What users said about focus groups.

- useful for developing staff skills that subsequently can be used internally for other purposes, for example, facilitation
- can be used to tackle other Health and Safety issues – helped us rethink our approach to clinical waste management
- there was a lack of participation by managers; they think it's an important issue but can't give time to it
- feeling is that despite difficulties the focus group approach has worked well and feedback from staff has been very good.

When planning focus groups:

- maintain commitment and momentum, plan to run focus groups as soon as possible after undertaking a survey
- the number, size and make up of focus groups will depend on local circumstances, for example, the issues that have been raised, the different groups of employees in the workplace and what is feasible and practicable
- typically a focus group should last no more that one and a half to two hours
- as much advanced notice as possible should be given to people attending
- consider how expectations can be managed; both for those attending the focus group and those that are not
- consider the location for focus groups – will participants be free from interruptions, comfortable and able to see/hear each other easily?
- an independent facilitator will be needed to lead the focus group. Their role is to set the scene, establish ground rules including confidentiality, topics for discussion, timekeeping, individual contributions and recording. The facilitator can be from another part of the organisation, but avoid appointing managers who may be perceived as part of the problem. It may be desirable to appoint a specialist or external facilitator, although with some training, anyone who is perceived as a good listener and with no 'axe to grind' can fulfil the role
- consider whether participants are likely to be comfortable expressing their honest opinions in front of each other. Aim for groups likely to face similar issues or who will have a common outlook. Avoid groups that are likely to be incompatible and also avoid bringing supervisors/managers together with junior grades, who may feel inhibited
- focus groups might begin with some general discussions around 'What is good/bad about working here?' (Acknowledge but agree to 'park' difficult issues beyond their control and remit)
- make progress on the good practice outlined in the 'states to be achieved' of the management standards. If the HSE survey has been used the results may lead to focusing on particular states or standards
- some issues may fit under more than one standard. Exploring this may help tease out what is the underlying problem – is it really workload for example or could employees cope with the work if support systems were better?
- remember to ask for ideas to improve the situation – this will be important when making a local action plan to tackle stress

- keep written notes of what people say to help prioritise and review in the future. An assistant to keep notes enables the facilitator to facilitate
- write up a summary as soon as possible after the focus group and send it to participants explaining how it will be used
- when analysing focus group summaries look for common themes and surprises. Tone and context are also important – did a particular comment trigger an emotional response or a number of comments?
- when writing the final report, take into account relevant context for example other sources of information such as surveys. Highlight the main themes, issues and questions that arose and how they will be addressed and prioritise these. Consider what can be tackled locally and what needs to be done at a wider level
- continue to use existing methods to discuss with employees issues that affect them at work, for example regular staff meetings, toolbox talks, or performance reviews.

Box 11.10 Some examples of questions for focus groups.

1 How does this match up to your experience? – *Key question.*
2 How do we know when the balance is right? – *Open question.*
3 How could improvements be made? – *Open question.*
4 Could you give me an example? – *Probing question.*
5 Does the rest of the group agree? – *Closed question.*
6 How well does that capture what we've said? – *Summary question.*

Further guidance on how to run focus groups is available to download from the HSE website[22] www.hse.gov.uk/stress/standards/pdfs/focusgroups.pdf.

Step 4: action planning

Having identified areas of concern and taken steps to develop solutions it is important to record the findings. The best method of achieving this is to write and disseminate an action plan.

An action plan will help set goals to work towards, facilitate prioritisation, demonstrate that employees' concerns are being taken seriously and provide a benchmark to evaluate and review against.

An action plan should at least include the following:

- what the problem is
- how the problem was identified
- what is being done in response
- how the solution was arrived at
- key milestones and dates for them to be reached
- commitment to provide feedback to employees on progress
- date for reviewing against the plan.

There is no prescribed method or format for an action plan. However, there are some good examples of what various organisations have done and a template that can be used on the HSE website. An in-depth case study is included later in this chapter including a summary of the key actions taken.

The action plan needs to be agreed with senior management and employee representatives and shared with employees. Consider carefully how best to do this. For example, if an intervention was popular in focus groups but is not practicable, you need to explain this. It is also important to communicate the implementation plan and outcome monitoring. Poor communication at this stage can quickly undermine the whole process.

Box 11.11 Further comments from users.

- There is no 'silver bullet' for stress
- Try and align with existing initiatives; don't reinvent the wheel
- It is often the small things that make the difference
- Once we agreed that the management standards must be incorporated into every day work it worked well
- We reintroduced regular team meetings to address workload, local cover and other immediate issues
- The Trust now expects managers to thank staff.

Step 5: monitor and review the effectiveness of interventions

It will be necessary to monitor and review any action taken to tackle stress. There are two elements to this:

1 monitor against the action plan periodically to check that agreed actions are being undertaken, for example that meetings are being held, or that there is evidence that certain activities have taken place
2 evaluate the effectiveness of the solutions implemented.

The method of evaluating the effectiveness of solutions is dependent upon the kind of solutions which have been developed. Use the SMART principle for evaluation.

It is important to ask those involved whether they feel the solutions are having the desired effect. It may only be necessary to check with a sample of those involved. Alternatively, it may be important to ensure that the intervention is working for everyone.

Another way to demonstrate the effectiveness of the plan is to collect data on employee turnover, sickness absence and productivity, measuring progress against emerging trends or changes in this data.

The timing of reviews is dependent on how long it takes to implement each intervention and how long the focus group expects it will take to have any impact. This could be days for a simple intervention, such as an adjustment to the physical environment, or months for piloting a complicated long-term solution such as a new rostering system.

Follow-up activity

The HSE recommends repeating the process on a regular basis perhaps every twelve to eighteen months or when significant change is planned.

Learning points

'One off' interventions or initiatives may not bring about sustainable improvements. The management standards approach is about making steady and continuous improvements in the way that stress is managed. It is critical to remain committed to a rolling programme of improvement, monitoring and review.

At the outset of this process managers often assume that when asking what the problems are and how they can be addressed, staff will ask for more resources. In the HSE's experience, this fear has not been borne out in practice. Most interventions are small and can be achieved with little or no extra cost. Many of the problems identified are failings in existing policies and procedures; things that should already be happening but for various reasons are not. These are often small things that slowly 'wind people up' and are perceived by staff as an indication that the organisation is failing to support employees.

The role of managers in the process is important. The key message is that policies and procedures are a starting point but are meaningless without the co-operation and support of managers at all levels of the organisation.

Finally, proactive management of stress is closely associated with good management practice and sound management techniques generally. Wherever possible, try to integrate as many of the principles or features of the process into everyday management practice. This will help sustain the gains made and minimise the need to repeat the process. Ultimately it will result in an improvement in the management culture of the organisation.

Will the HSE enforce the management standards?

The HSE has already served a small number of Improvement Notices for failure to make a suitable and sufficient assessment of the risks to the health and safety of employees from exposure to work related stressors. Most notable was that served against West Dorset General Hospitals NHS Trust in 2003.[23] The Trust complied with the notice by adopting a management standards-based approach.

More recently, the HSE has turned its attention to providing advice and support on performing risk assessments for work-related stress, rather than a traditional enforcement-led approach. The management standards are currently set out as guidance because when they were being developed the HSC took the view that regulations or an ACOP were not appropriate. This was because there was insufficient evidence regarding prevention and management of workplace stressors. The nature of stress means a 'one size fits all' approach is clearly not appropriate so the HSE developed a flexible process.

The HSE promotes voluntary uptake of the management standards. However, in the future the enforcement strategy will be reviewed. The HSE may then look to take action against those who show clear disregard for the health risks posed to their employees by work-related stress.

Using the management standards approach is one way for organisations to show that they are meeting, or working towards meeting, their legal obligation to tackle work-related stress.

Are other approaches acceptable?

There may be alternative approaches thought to be more suitable for some organisations' needs. There is no requirement to use the HSE Management

Standards. However, based on the available evidence, the HSE view is that an effective organisational approach to tackling work-related stress should include:

- collecting a range of information on the current situation – such as sickness absence, staff turnover or by using staff surveys
- promoting active discussion with employees and trade unions to identify how the information translates locally and working in partnership to make practical improvements
- agreeing and sharing an action plan with staff
- regularly reviewing the situation to ensure continued improvement.

What is HSE doing to promote use of the standards?

There is a programme of education and training available for managers and staff to increase awareness of what stress is and its consequences if not properly managed. Work is underway with organisations from five sectors that report the highest levels of workplace stress. Supporting these organisations as they implement the management standards is providing a rich source of case study material[24] and practical advice on what works well and what doesn't. Using this information, the HSE has rolled out a programme of practical workshops around the country to encourage use of the management standards.

Website material is continually updated to reflect the latest thinking in this area. The HSE is funding research into the management competencies[25] needed to effectively implement the Management Standards in order to facilitate links with the HR agenda. There is joint working with key stakeholders – professional bodies, training providers, Government departments – to promote the approach and influence the debate around stress in the workplace, which in turn links with initiatives such as 'Good Jobs'[26] and 'Health, Work and Well-being'.[27]

By continuing to raise awareness of the issues and promoting a proactive approach to stress management, the HSE will continue to help organisations make real and measurable progress towards improving the modern working environment and the health and well-being of their employees.

Box 11.12 Some final comments from users.

- This has been a positive experience for all involved
- This has been a really interesting, exciting, worthwhile process. it has also been hard work and frustrating at times
- We have already seen an increase in staff motivation
- We should encourage others to do it – an excellent approach.

Case study: application of the HSE management standards at Hinchingbrooke Healthcare NHS Trust

Background

Hinchingbrooke Healthcare NHS Trust comprises Hinchingbrooke Hospital, an acute general hospital in Cambridgeshire with 342 beds, a busy A&E department and high volumes of day surgery, out-patient and diagnostic work. The hospital employs 1,800 staff.

The Healthcare Commission awarded the Trust a zero-star rating in 2002 after which the newly appointed management team and their Chief Executive Officer (CEO) initiated a performance improvement plan. The Trust was awarded two stars – out of a possible three – in 2003, which it retained in 2004 and 2005.

Why a stress management initiative?

In 2003 there was a growing feeling of stress amongst staff. As the director of HR and Communications put it 'the "S" word was taking on a life of its own – it was the new buzz word'. Two attacks on staff at the hospital led to serious alarm, following which the HSE issued an Improvement Notice in relation to security and staff safety. Occupational health saw an increase in stress related illnesses and the 2003 NHS national employee attitude survey found that Hinchingbrooke was in the 20% of Trusts with the highest degree of work pressure felt by staff. There was a perception that middle management acted as a 'damp proof course' inhibiting both downward and upward communication flows.

At West Dorset General Hospitals NHS Trust in July 2003, following complaints about bullying and long working hours, an HSE inspection found that there was no stress policy in place and no risk assessment for work related stress. The HSE served an Improvement Notice.

The West Dorset case was the catalyst that enabled Hinchingbrooke's CEO to call for urgent action on stress management, with the enthusiastic support of trade unions and staff. The HR director and occupational health nurse manager – both relatively new to the Trust – worked together to devise and manage the initiative.

Hinchingbrooke's employee assistance programme provider was asked to report on work related issues that were contributing to stress. The occupational health nurse manager produced a report to the Trust Board, detailing the case for action and suggesting the way forward, which was agreed. In November the CEO published an article to all staff putting stress on the agenda. His article included the following passages:

> As we all work harder to achieve more, it is inevitable that we will feel the strain and the pressure of work will increase. None of us is exempt from feeling, at times, that it is becoming more difficult to cope.
>
> We will be looking at sources of stress within the Trust and drawing up an action plan for addressing these where possible. This project will involve staff at all levels as we make a concerted effort to reduce stress by tackling its sources.

The 2004 diagnostic survey

In early 2004 the HSE published its draft Management Standards on Work Related Stress,[28] launched in their final form later that year. The six Standards – Demands, Control, Support, Relationships, Role, Change – aimed to provide a workplace with high levels of employee well-being and minimal stress.

The Trust wanted an 'on-line' employee survey questionnaire that would:

- measure the Trust's true levels of stress against all of the HSE Standards
- identify which areas of the Trust were performing well and which were suffering the most
- use the HSE benchmark percentages as a guide to the Trust's performance
- provide a fast turn round of results to meet staff expectations.

The NHS national employee attitude survey designed by Aston University, which is administered annually to all Trusts, was used for the first time in the previous year. The national survey did not contain questions covering all six Standards, and those that were covered were not investigated with a sufficient range of questions to be fully HSE compliant. Trusts can add their own questions to the national survey, but it was decided to opt for a separate survey,[29] designed specifically around the HSE stress standards.

The selected survey offered:

- HSE benchmarked and compliant
- allowed for an unlimited number of optional extra demographic questions agreed at the outset, enabling the data to be sorted and reported to the organisation's specification in terms of business unit, job function, job grade and demographic group. Hinchingbrooke selected the demographic categorisations used in the national NHS (Aston) survey
- the questionnaire was sent electronically as one e-mail to all employees' e-mail addresses. Paper copies were sent to staff with no e-mail account, people on longer-term absence such as those on maternity leave and to staff who had not responded
- the questionnaire took six minutes to complete. Staff with e-mail addresses completed the questionnaire on line to an external website, with the data stored and analysed on an external server. This meant that several people could enter their responses at once, staff were assured that their answers were confidential and the external provider undertook all analysis automatically
- the reporting methodology used traffic lights adopting the HSE convention. Comparing the organisation's performance with the HSE benchmark data (the scores of a nationally representative sample of nearly 2,000 employees collected in 2004).

The traffic light codings used were:

- **green doing very well – need to maintain** represents results in or close to the top 20% of the scores of the national benchmark sample
- **blue good – but need for improvement** represents results better than average but not yet in or close to the benchmark top 20%
- **amber – clear need for improvement** represents results below average but not in or close to the bottom benchmark 20%
- **red – urgent action needed** represents results in or close to the bottom benchmark 20%.

The reporting tool suggested targets for improvement using an HSE methodology. Each of the six management standards was investigated through several questions. Thus, demands were reported in four elements:

1 do you have to work excessively fast?
2 do you have to work very intensively?
3 do you have enough time to do everything?

4 do different groups at work demand things from you that you think are hard to combine?

An external provider trained Hinchingbrooke staff to generate reports and queries from the server database and additionally offered the option of supplying the data as an Excel spreadsheet from which Trust staff could generate reports.

The Trust administered the survey, giving staff three weeks to respond together with an extra week's grace for late returns. There was a problem when it emerged that 400 staff e-mail accounts were for staff who had either left or had never accessed their e-mail with the result that their in-boxes were full. After the redundant e-mail accounts had been discounted the response rate was above 80%.

Table 11.1 Survey results for Hinchingbrooke Healthcare NHS Trust.

HSE standard (with HSE benchmark)	July 2004 survey	July 2005 survey	Comments
Demands (85%)	20%	60%	Huge improvement. Particularly strong improvement in feelings of having to work long hours and deadlines being unachievable
Control (85%)	65%	72%	Step in right direction – links with demands
Support (85%)	85%	76%	Issues on support from manager rather than peer group
Relationships (65%)	75%	76%	Improvement
Role (65%)	70%	84%	Superb
Change (65%)	70%	64%	Scale of change going on

▨ Red   ▨ Orange   ▨ Green

Results were reported for the Trust as a whole (see Table 11.1), for each associate director's area and for each of the pre-selected demographic and functional staff groups. For the Trust as a whole demands were coded red (urgent action needed), with control at amber (clear need for improvement). Discussion with the HSE showed that the two were linked; giving staff increased control would help the management of demands.

The reporting for each associate director's area flagged up areas for attention specific to each. Staff in one department felt bullied, suggesting that the department head's management style needed adjustment through sensitive counselling and coaching.

The Trust was clear that feedback to staff was key. The survey results were communicated promptly in a process managed by the communications manager. The timetable was:

- July: survey
- August: results presented to the Trust Board with positive points and issues needing attention. Tabletop A5 flyers and posters across the Trust including the

library and restaurant areas, with three key success messages and three areas for improvement

- September: three-page booklet for all staff, explaining the issues. Time to 'quiz' the HR director in the staff restaurant. Article in the staff magazine
- October: opportunity to discuss with HR and senior managers.

The report for each managerial area was sent out individually to the relevant Associate Director to discuss with staff, collect their ideas for action and submit an action plan within one month. The actions were sometimes as simple as setting up monthly staff meetings.

The 'valuing staff' campaign

The Trust delivered a 'Valuing Staff' campaign over the following year with the involvement and support of staff trade unions. The campaign was publicised at the outset by a stand outside the staff dining room set up and staffed by occupational health. Initiatives were progressed in nine key areas:

1 Written guidance to managers and staff.
- The 'Policy for Managing Work Related Stress and Psychological Well Being in the Workplace' set out the Trust's approach and detailed the responsibilities of the Trust at corporate level, managers, employees, occupational health, HR, safety representatives and the Health and Safety Committee.
- The key message is that psychological well-being should be approached at different levels. At the corporate level to develop policies and processes to minimise the risk occurring and at the management level to provide leadership and good management practices that encourage team working and good communication between individuals and their managers. At an individual level to recognise the nature and causes of stress and to manage stress effectively by aiming to achieve a good work-life balance.
- A booklet 'Managing Stress at Work: Support for Managers and Staff', covering what is stress, how to recognise stress, managing stress and sources of support.
2 The Trust acted to better predict patient demand and to provide appropriate staffing levels from day-to-day.
- An algorithm was developed to predict A&E attendances. This proved highly successful in enabling managers to match staffing to demand in the A&E department and in emergency admissions wards.
- Elective admissions for planned work proved to be less hard to predict. So the Trust re-designed the processes, moving as much surgery as possible to day case or 23 hour stay work so reducing demand on in-patient beds and building more predictability into the system.
- Middle managers re-deployed staff from one ward to another from day-to-day in order to take account of the number of staff available for duty at the beginning of each shift.
3 Every job advertised had a recently reviewed job description and candidate specification, followed by careful recruitment and selection, to ensure 'right person, right job'.
4 The Trust promoted a warm, appreciative and participative management style. In particular the Trust expected managers to thank staff measured by a

question in the annual stress survey. The Trust's comments on the 2005 survey result included 'whilst managers are approachable, the amount of positive praise and feedback has fallen – are we saying thank you enough?'

5 The Trust expected that everyone would have a quality annual Performance Development Review meeting with his/her manager. Joint objective setting in the meeting generating SMART job targets and personal development plans, supported by routine one to one meetings over the year to track progress and identify problems.

6 The Trust worked to ensure that appropriate work life balance options were available to everyone needing them.

7 The Trust delivered a communication strategy to ensure that all employees were kept informed. This had three strands:

- the CEO held monthly 'walkabout' meetings, at which he addressed staff and discussed current issues. The time and location varied from month to month to improve staff access. The 'Improving Working Lives Practice Plus' report found that these 'are highly valued by staff and promote good communications'
- all managers held monthly one-hour briefing group meetings with their staff, which proved very successful and offered opportunities for staff to discuss issues and to input to decision making
- the Trust published 'Challenging Times', a weekly staff newsletter with the brand 'if it's not in "Challenging Times", it's not true', and its monthly staff magazine 'Pulse'.

8 Effective attendance management was made a mandatory requirement for all managers to maximise staffing levels on the ground and to support staff. The Trust expected managers to:

- pick up early signs
- encourage use of the Trust's employee assistance programme, which provided a 24 hour telephone advice service as well as face to face counselling
- refer to occupational health at the earliest opportunity. Occupational health to meet with the member of staff to:
    - identify any ongoing medical issues
    - explore the perceived causes of stress, using the HSE standards approach to identify the work related factors, that is, role and demands which were causing the problem. This had the additional benefit of preventing other members of the same team suffering similar problems
    - advise the employee and manager to work through the HSE Standards and develop solutions
    - ensure that the member of staff received appropriate treatment and support.
- keep in regular touch with the member of staff whilst off sick, particularly in the case of long term absence
- manage the person's return to work – as the Trust put it, 'think Walker'.[30] The line manager should:
    - meet the person *before* their return to work to ensure that any workplace stressors are identified
    - discuss a rehabilitation plan with occupational health
    - conduct a risk assessment by reviewing the job description, person

specification and the member of staff's skills and aptitudes, and review to identify whether any additional changes are needed – Demands, Control, Support, Relationships, Role, Change
  – conduct a return to work interview.
* Ensure that any agreed support mechanisms are actioned and monitor how well these are working.

Managers were supported by a booklet published by the organisation Mind Out for Mental Health, entitled the 'Line Managers' Resource: a practical guide to managing and supporting mental health in the workplace'.[31] Providing practical advice on managing and supporting people experiencing stress, distress and mental health problems. The booklet can be downloaded from the Mindful Employer website.

9 These initiatives required managers to take 'ownership' of managing their staff, so the Trust invested heavily in management development. The Trust identified education as the keystone. The process started in with one-day workshops on the use of transactional analysis to develop impact and influence. The Trust went on to introduce two courses run 'in house' but accredited by the Institute of Leadership and Management:
* the Core Management Skills programme an introductory course
* the Essential Management Skills programme to develop management skills further, operating as a five day block with two subsequent days. The Trust's subsequent 'Improving Working Lives Practice Plus' report found the programme 'immensely popular and effective.' The course included a half day session on how to manage stress at work and covered the nature and causes of stress, national and local incidence, the Trust's stress policy and its implementation and the role of occupational health.

Counselling and coaching help was made available for managers needing support.
   The management development programme was made a requirement for new managers and for managers on promotion and other managers who volunteered to participate were found places. The next step was to identify the management development needs of all existing managers through the appraisal process and in the context of the NHS Key Skills Framework and to deliver appropriate management development for everyone.

Outcomes – the results for Hinchingbrooke

* Staff sickness absence was down from 6% to 3.8% giving the hospital one of the lowest NHS absence rates in the UK. The Trust estimated that this has reduced the cost of agency cover by £500,000 each year.
* The Trust repeated the stress survey the following year. The repeat survey showed huge improvement in terms of demands and progress on control. The support score had slipped back, reflecting a need for managers to be more attentive to the support needs of staff.
* The Trust was awarded 'Improving Working Lives Practice Plus' status, the highest level of award in the NHS for HR.
* In the national NHS staff survey prior to the initiative Hinchingbrooke was in the 20% of Trusts with the highest degree of work pressure felt by staff. The hospital subsequently moved into the lowest 20%. The same survey found that the number of staff with intention to leave had fallen.

- The hospital's employer brand improved, evidenced by movement from a range of unfilled health care assistant vacancies to a waiting list of applicants.
- The number of reports of stress had gone up, possibly reflecting greater awareness of the issue and willingness to seek help.
- Productivity has substantially increased, including reductions in waiting times, the opening of a major new facility for diagnostic work and day surgery with increasing patient throughput.

Hinchingbrooke's achievement was particularly strong given a background of ward closures to save money. In March 2006 the Trust announced a further planned 10% saving in staff costs, a major test of the hospital's ability to manage its staff successfully through major turbulence.

Cost benefit

Significant investments in the initiative were in management development and in funding half the time of the occupational health nurse manager for the first six months whilst she developed and launched the programme. The audit tool used by the Trust was low cost, the expense of additional internal communications was absorbed by existing budgets.

Ongoing expenditure is expected to be the cost of management development and a quarter of the time of an occupational health nurse for case management and participation in delivering management development.

These investments delivered a saving of £500,000 per annum in agency cover together with increasing productivity. The effort put into the stress management initiative also went a long way towards enabling the Trust to achieve a range of other objectives, including:

- meeting NHS Key Performance Indicator targets for acute Trusts, including managing demand particularly in A&E
- achieving the standards set in the NHS Trust Performance Management Framework or 'annual health check' launched in Spring 2005, particularly in relation to Safety and Governance
- earning the award of 'Improving Working Lives Practice Plus' status.

Evaluation of the initiative

Managers at the Trust reflected that management commitment and skill, workforce participation and excellent communications were all key to success.

A five-year programme was needed to achieve cultural change. In addition skilled management acting on the style and people management policies of the Trust dealt promptly with problems of performance.

There could have been greater monitoring of associate directors' areas to ensure that each one generated an action plan in discussion with staff after each survey and that the actions were delivered. This might have involved HR presenting the action plans to the Board together with six monthly progress reports covering both corporate and directorate actions. There might have been more work to educate managers and staff in depth from the outset, using 'guest spots' in existing forums. Planned sessions on stress could usefully have been incorporated in the annual training and development calendar.

Conclusion

'Staff have to be happy, healthy and here, that is at work, in order to deliver efficiency gains and first rate services. That is the best way to position our organisations to better deliver core functions.'

Lord Hunt of King's Heath,
Ministerial Task Force on Health, Safety and Productivity.

'Buzz' words and initiatives come and go. What the HSE is aiming to achieve through promoting the management standards approach is a more fundamental change in management culture – it's not enough to carry out a risk assessment for stress then file it and forget about it until the inspector calls. The emphasis is on actions; the challenge to managers is:

What are you doing to make your workplace a healthy one? And how do you know it is working?

References

1 Health and Safety Executive: Management Standards. www.hse.gov.uk/stress/ standards.
2 NHS Employer website: www.nhsemployers.org.
3 Managing Sickness Absence in the Public Sector. A joint review by the Ministerial Task Force for Health, Safety and Productivity and the Cabinet Office. November 2004. Available at: www.hse.gov.uk/gse/sickness.pdf (last accessed 20/11/2006).
4 NHS Partners: *Sickness absence and staff turnover.* August 2005.
5 The Information Centre for health and social care. Sickness absence rates of NHS Staff in 2005. May 2006. Available at: www.ic.nhs.uk/pubs/sicknessabsencerates.
6 Health and Safety Executive. *Securing Health Together: A long-term occupational health strategy for England, Scotland and Wales.* MISC225. London: HSE Books; 2000.
7 Strategy statement: the Department of the Environment, Transport and the Regions. *Revitalising Health and Safety.* HMSO: London; 2000.
8 Health and Safety Executive. *Real Solutions; Real People: a managers' guide to tackling work-related stress.* London: HSE Books; 2003
9 Healthcare Commission. National Survey of NHS Staff 2005. March 2006. Available at: www.healthcarecommission.org.uk/nationalfindings/surveys/staffsurveys/2005nhsstaffsurvey.cfm.
10 Healthcare Commission. Survey of Inpatients 2005. March 2006. Available at: www.healthcarecommission.org.uk/nationalfindings/surveys/patientsurveys/nhspatientsurvey2005/inpatientsurvey2005.cfm.
11 Health and Safety Executive. *Tackling work-related stress - a managers' guide to improving and maintaining employee health and well-being.* HSG218 2001. HSE Books; (currently out of print). Note: a revised publication is due mid 2007 which will replace both HSG218 and Real Solutions; Real People.
12 Jones J, Huxtable C, Hodgson J. Self Reported work-related illness in 2004/05: Results from the Labour Force Survey. November 2006. Available at: http://www.hse.gsi.gov.uk/statistics.
13 Health and Safety Executive. *Managing Stress at Work: Discussion document* DDE10 C150. London: HSE Books; 1999.
14 Health and Safety at Work Act 1974. London: HMSO; 1974.
15 Health and Safety Executive. *Management of Health and Safety at Work Regulations 1999. Approved Code of Practice and guidance.* L21.London: HSE Books; 2000.

16 Health and Safety Executive. Managing sickness absence and return to work. Good practice guidance is available at: www.hse.gov.uk/sicknessabsence/index.htm.

17 Health and Safety Executive. 5 steps to risk assessment. INDG 163 (rev2). HSE Books; 2006. Available at: www.hse.gov.uk/risk/fivesteps.htm.

18 Kelly C, Mellor N. Evaluation of the Management Standards pilot study Health and Safety Laboratory. Report no. WPS/04/05 (unpublished).

19 MacKay C, Cousins R, Kelly P, *et al*. Management Standards and work-related stress in the UK: Policy background and science. *Work & Stress*. 2004; **18**(2): 91–112.

20 Cousins R, MacKay C, Clarke S. *et al*. Management Standards and work-related stress in the UK: Practical Development. *Work & Stress*. 2004; **18**(2): 113–6.

21 Health and Safety Executive. Psychosocial Working Conditions in Britain in 2004. London: HSE; 2004.

22 Health and Safety Executive. How to organise and run focus groups. Available at: www.hse.gov.uk/stress/standards/pdfs/focusgroups.pdf.

23 Health and safety offences and penalties 2003/04 – industry examples: Work-related stress in the NHS. Case study available at: http://www.hse.gov.uk/enforce/off03–04/examples.htm#4 (last accessed 20/11/06).

24 Case studies are available on HSE's website at: http://www.hse.gov.uk/stress/experience.htm.

25 Donaldson-Fielder E, Pryce J, Lewis R. *Stress Management Competence: Identifying and developing the management behaviours necessary to implement the HSE management standards*. London: HSE; 2005.

26 The Work Foundation and the London Health Commission. Healthy Work: Productive Workplaces. Why the UK needs more 'good jobs'. December 2005. Available at: http://www.theworkfoundation.com/products/publications/azpublications/healthywo rkproductiveworkplaceswhytheukneedsmoregoodjobs.aspx.

27 Department for Work and Pensions, the Department of Health and the Health and Safety Executive. Health, Work and Well-being – caring for our future: a strategy for the health and well-being of working age people. HM Government 2005. Available at: www.dwp.gov.uk/publications/dwp/2005/health_and_wellbeing.pdf (last accessed 20/11/06).

28 Management Standards consultation exercise 2004. Summary of responses and final report on the consultation available at: http://www.hse.gov.uk/consult/condocs/stressms.htm (last accessed 20/11/06).

29 www.stresswatch.net.

30 Walker v. Northumberland County Council 1995 1 All ER 737.

31 A practical guide to managing and supporting mental health in the workplace: line managers' resource. Available to download from the Mindful Employer website at: www.mindfulemployer.net/Line%20Managers%20Resource.pdf.

Further reading

- HSE website.
- Real Solutions, Real People: A managers' guide to tackling work-related stress. London: HSE Books; 2003.
- Risk Management: work and organisational Factors. *Work and Stress*. 2004; **18**(2): 89–185.

Index